In Case I Forget

The Story

OF A

LEWY BODY SOLDIER

Forward

The first I knew of the Purple Angel was sitting in the doctors' waiting room with mum, who has vascular dementia and seeing a message on the television screen about a memory cafe at Barton Baptist Church, Barton, in Devon.

I had moved to Devon to look after mum after dad had passed away and was finding life extremely difficult. So I decided to go along and see what it was like. The best decision I had made in a very long while! I haven't looked back since and have become friends with Norrms and Elaine.

Norrms is an inspiration, not only to me, but with all he meets. His passion for fighting against this awful disease, Dementia, and trying to get the best done to improve the lives for all who suffer, including the carers, is amazing. Once he gets the bit between the teeth, no-one can stop him.

As I have known him for a couple of years now, I realise just how hard he and Elaine have to fight to battle the many challenges in changes to his own health. I often wonder how they do what they do. I do know why, he tells me often enough!

It is with great respect and admiration, both for him and Elaine, that I call myself their friend. We spend a lot of time together and have such a lot of fun and laughter, I cannot imagine a time when this may come to an end. I know Norrms is not feeling as well as he could do, but he continues to face each day head on with strength and courage. The title of his book is so apt and I will always remember the Lewy Body's Soldier. X

Dedication

I first met Norrms at one of his early meetings; I was there because my wife has Alzheimer's. I immediately saw how dedicated and determined he was to get Dementia recognised, making people aware of Dementia for what it is, an illness. It has been through his resolve as someone with Dementia that he achieved so much in a short time. His suggested name, the Purple Angel was immediately adopted worldwide and will be his lasting legacy. His Dementia Diary, a Sunday morning broadcast on BBC Devon and now this book will continue to make everyone aware of this dreadful illness that affects so many.

We must not forget his wife Elaine who he calls his Angel and who does so much to support him and, was the inspiration for the name, Purple Angel.

I am pleased to have Norrms as a friend, above all though, he is a friend of all Dementia suffers,

Ted Tuckerman.

Being EIGHT years into my diagnosis of dementia this will be my last book. It scares me to death to say such a thing but facts are facts, and if they don't find a cure very soon, the inevitable will happen for sure. Truth be known, It should have happened years ago, and if it wasn't for the love, dedication and sheer strength given to me by my lifelong Partner Elaine, who is also the reason why the PURPLE ANGEL has her name, as she truly is an Angel who walks this earth and has kept me safe all these years, I wouldn't be here now writing this book.

I also have to say a HUGE thank you to Co-founder or the Purple Angel Campaign Jane Moore who has been by mine and Elaine's side ALL through the ups and downs , successes and failures and yet still put up with us, you are one in a million my friend

A HUGE THANK YOU TO The steering group of the Torbay Dementia Action Alliance, who have also stuck by me through thick and thin, and certainly kept me in my place as chairperson are as follows, and In NO particular Order loll

Roz Jupp, Lisa Doran, Sam Ebden, Elaine Waddingham, Bridie Moorehouse, Carolyn Starkins, Stephanie Janka Spurlock, Phillip and Lorraine Hutchins (or will be soon!) Bob Jope, Liz Kirkpatrick, Amanda martin, Julie Reshard

Regrets? A few, but if I had my time over again, I wouldn't hesitate in searching Elaine out and doing it all AGAIN!! How many can say that!!!

WEBSITE

http://www.purpleangel-global.com/

TDAA WEBSITE

http://tdaa.global/

Chapter one

OH NO NOT AGAIN!!!

Why is the radio on as well as the television I asked? "It's not" replied Elaine "why, what can you hear? " I can hear someone else talking; it sounds like they are behind me"

Just then, a dark shadow ran in front of me fleetingly and darted off at speed, disappearing before my very eyes. The shock on my face told Elaine I had just seen something awful, and yet she hadn't, this was how it all started, this was when we knew Lewy Body`s had come to call ....

My nightmares soon turned into Night terrors, so totally different, and then came the hallucinations. Because Elaine has 30 years + in care work, once again she knew something wasn't right and an appointment was made to go back and see the specialist, thankfully, a different specialist.

Someone once said they couldn't imagine anything worse than being told you have dementia. I now know there is, and that's being told you have dementia TWICE!! I had spent FOUR LONG years reading up, learning and trying to understand Alzheimer's disease, all aspects from beginning to end.

I believed that you wouldn't go to war without knowing your enemy, so why would I NOT learn as much as I could about it, only to be told they were wrong, and it was actually Lewy Body's dementia I had. YEP!! I had to start all over again!!! Lewy Body's is so different to Alzheimer's as I will try to explain later on in the book (All in my own opinion as I am not medically trained) it was still as devastating as being told the first time. The specialist who came to see us had just moved down to Devon from Newcastle and was involved in the very early stages of research into Lewy body's, so if one can 'feel lucky' about being diagnosed with dementia, I suppose it was me, but only 'lucky' in the fact we had not only a specialist in his field, but also a specialist in Lewy body's Type Dementia.

Since that day when he dropped the bombshell of my second diagnosis, a lot of what I was doing began to make a little sense (little being the operative word) but at least it did, and from that day I knew I had to start all over again and once more GO TO WAR with yet another enemy, only this time it was called Lewy Body's and not Alzheimer's. The thought of trying to do it all again had me so worried as I knew I wasn't any better in myself than I was four years ago, I was actually a little worse, but as always, with the help of my family and friends rallying around me and helping me all they could. We spent hours, trawling the internet, contacting Lewy body's Society UK and finding out as much as we could.

What we did find out TOTALLY shocked me!! And not just the intricacies of the disease either! I could not believe what a HUGE chasm, information and help wise, there was between types of dementias, I was absolutely flummoxed as to why MOST people I came across had never even heard of Lewy body's (something that has haunted me ever since and still does I may add!!) How can this be?? How can many people just think there is one type of dementia only? I have to say at this point it's nobody's fault, you 'Don't Know' what you 'Don't Know' until you are told, but it's hard to believe that. The lack of information and help that was out there for what is a terminal disease was so very poor. The more I learned about how bad it was out there, the more I realised so many people were just about getting by with little or no help regarding this type of disease.

Some of the information I found could end up being possibly life threatening. I found out that in some cases, if you didn't give the right medication to those with Lewy Body's and give them medication that's designed for other types of dementia it could have very serious consequences!!

Now, is this just me being pedantic, or is it common sense? Would you give someone who has heart problems medication that relieved those symptoms and not give them medication for, say, Liver failure or Shingles?? WHY on God's green earth doesn't the same apply to Dementia??? We know it doesn't in some cases and the results can be catastrophic. I find it very hard to believe that this goes on but we have met too many people to say it doesn't. This is just one of many things that need to change. I have met so many people who I have asked "What type of dementia have you?" Many replied Alzheimer's, and yet when we discuss symptoms, it appears so many of them have the same symptoms as me. This is something that has niggled me for years, and the reason I have challenged this time and time again, as yet with no adequate answer as far as I'm concerned, I will carry on asking these questions, and many more, until we all get the satisfactory answers we require. Some say 'It's not as simple as that' the thing is, it can be if you want it to be, here's an example ……………………

Shortly after being re-diagnosed I did a presentation in a nearby Devon coastal town. It was one of the few I have done where Drs, Gods ERRR sorry I mean Consultants (LOL) were present as well as carers and people living with dementia. I stood on stage, knowing how many professionals were there and asked the question , please raise your hand's if you know……………

"What are the signs of Early Dementia?"

Hands shot up in the air quicker than you could blink!!! And mostly from the Gps etc. In turn they answered, 'Forgetfulness, Confusion, Spatial awareness, Disorientation,' and many more, and, ALL CORRECT I MAY ADD!!

Unknown to them all, I had done my homework, as I then asked "If that's the case, and you ALL know the early signs of dementia , why then, is there are only 67 people in the town we sit, diagnosed with dementia??? Either it's the best place in the World to live, OR there is something very wrong I said!!!" The room fell deathly quiet; there were rustlings and shifting movements on their chairs as a look of both confusion and guilt spread across their faces. Suddenly, one of the GP`s blurted out those immortal words 'It's not as simple as that'. I was, as they say up North, GOBSMACKED!!

Hang on a minute I quickly said, if a person came into your surgery and informed you of chest pains you would think heart trouble. If a person came into your surgery and informed you of blinding headaches and nose bleeds you would think of Aneurysm. If someone came into your surgery and informed you of a persistent cough and rapid weight loss you would think possibly Cancer?

AND YET!! when someone comes into your surgery and they or their loved one/carer informs you of confusion, forgetfulness or spatial awareness you don't think DEMENTIA??
I have to say I didn't make many friends that day, and haven't been asked back since, strangely enough, but I do know, not long after, the diagnosis rate was a lot higher. Don't think for one minute it was because of me, but I do like to think I made them think, as I hope I have you?

I was devastated to be told I had dementia twice, and I was also LOST for a while as the 'Concrete overcoat' as I call it (depression) once again engulfed my mind and soul and dragged me down to the depths of despair.

But now, now I was once again on a mission. A mission to make sure as many people as possible knew there was more than just ONE TYPE of dementia; I wanted to make sure ALL understood that there were many types of dementia with many differing symptoms and medications needed for them. I wanted to make sure NOBODY slipped through the net of care and all got the best care they could.

A tall order I agree, but as I sat there, all sorts of ideas were running through my head.

We had, for the last four years been on a mission trying to educate people that this disease can happen to anybody, at any time, at any age, and wasn't just a disease of the elderly. I myself was diagnosed at just 50 years old. Both Elaine and I had fought for four years with authorities, especially housing and care companies who only saw the age and not the illness. They said no to housing and flats because we were not 55 and over??? These were people who said they cared for the sick, and yet had no policies in place for younger people who were diagnosed with Dementia regarding housing, respite and so much more. The good thing was, that at this time, things were beginning to change, and change for the better when it came to those who have dementia and of course their carer`s. Movements were beginning, people were starting to stand up and talk out loud about dementia. It was starting to be discussed not only in Parliament, but on the streets, in homes and in workplaces.

Just over four years ago, from the date of writing this, was the first time I ever met David Cameron, Prime Minister of the United Kingdom for the very first time, it was going to be one of three incredible meetings that year with him which included a trip to Downing Street and having lunch with him and many others on the day, little knowing that when I was first diagnosed with Dementia and as far as I was concerned my life, as I knew it, would soon be over, would this be happening to me. That the path of life would lead me to a face to face meeting with him at the Russell Hotel in London, (literally face to face as I sat next to him!) and then onto Downing street, but it did. I knew then there was so much that was wrong, so much that needed doing and so much that had to be changed.

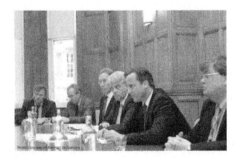

At this time I wanted change to happen there and then, if not before, but I soon came to realise that this wasn't going to happen overnight and many times I had to bite my tongue (as you can imagine), it was so incredibly frustrating. We soon realised how full the world is of red tape and people trying to stop you doing what you want to do, just because it wasn't 'PC'. We had lost faith in the old fashioned values of Common Sense and were all lost in a sea of 'Can I do this? Am I allowed to do that? What will people say if we do this without a RISK ASSESMENT???'

We had all fallen into this trap of self-doubt and lacking confidence in what we can actually do if we only realised that working together was the only way forward. I had no idea at the time how hard that last statement 'All Working Together' would be as we came up against barrier after barrier, and as one door closed, so did another!! But did it stop us? No! Did it make us give up? NO! Indeed not!

What it did do was make us more determined than ever to change things for the better, to try and improve services and condition's for both those living with dementia and their carer`s and to hopefully make sure that as many people as possible knew about every type of dementia, and not just one.

That was when the LEWY BODY SOLDIER was born! That was when we knew we had to do as much as possible to make sure people understood that there was life after diagnosis and try and make sure they knew that there were services out there that could get better with the right guidance and understanding. We knew we had such a HUGE battle ahead. We had so many plans, and yet, we had no idea how much time I had to do any of this. Forward we went anyway, into the unknown and with a new diagnosis. So much to do, so much to learn and so many new things to understand about Lewy body's Dementia, and remember, The Purple Angel campaign was still two years away from being just an idea, let alone becoming the force it is today.

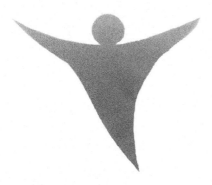

BLOG   >>>>>>>>>>>>>>>>>>>>>>>>>>>

Seems So Long Ago

As we turned the corner on the country road towards the garden centre, I put the radio on. Just starting to play was Mr Beau Jangles, one of my favourites. As I listened to how he had it all, how he sang and danced, and how, even now when all was lost he could still hear the crowd asking him to do more, I felt deflated as I realised how much we had in common.

My mind raced back as fast as light to a time where I would run into the disco, straight up to the DJ and ask for my favourite record (whatever it was at the time). I remember dancing away until my feet hurt, only stopping for light refreshment and to wipe my brow. I had forgotten how much I used to love to dance, how free I felt as I expressed myself in a way only I could!! (there`s a clue there LOL) and how the youthful blood used to run through my body as I jived, bopped and strutted my stuff to the tunes of the Top Twenty!!

Then I came back to earth with a THUD!! I remembered my illness of Dementia and my inability to remember most things, how it had stopped me from expressing myself, how it had stopped me being independent and going out to work to provide for my family as I had done for so many years. As I looked down at my hands they were white! Not because I was so cold but because I had clenched my fists so tight and was so frustrated!!! Where has it all gone?? WHY ME WHY ME? screamed through my head time after time. The noise in my head sounded like a platoon of marching soldiers as my blood pressure rose and just as I felt I was going to scream, we reached the top of the hill, and the view in front of me was OUTSTANDING!!!

I was looking up, towards Dartmoor, the rolling hills bathed in winter sunshine and yet tufts of snow were still visible right on the top of the highest hill. All around seemed so calm and surreal, and as I watched as the clouds cast it shadows across the moors only to be replaced by more rays of sunshine, did I begin to understand. Those dark clouds I had just seen casting their ugly shadows across the lush green fields are just the same as the mood that had just passed through my body and mind, only to be replaced by the warmth and brightness of the sun that breathed new life into my body and hope in my heart.

"We cannot bring the past back my friends, but we can bring the future forward"

CC Norrms Mc Namara

END OF BLOG   >>

CHAPTER TWO

The Lewy Body

Soldier

The name "The Lewy Body Soldier" is something I was called a while ago by a very good friend who lives in the town of Blackburn which is very near my home town of Bolton (you know who you are LOL xxx)

It's a very good way to explain things as you will see.

A soldier carries on and fights for what he thinks is right, he does his job no matter what and would risk all for family, Queen and country, never looking back, always forward and never giving up no matter what the odds were or how bad things got, always fighting, never retreating.

Sound familiar?? This applies to most people who have this awful disease, not just Lewy Body`s, but Dementia in general. We don't want to fight this war, but we have too!! We don't want to wake up each day knowing there is no end in sight to this daily battle and things will probably get worse before and 'IF' they get better, but we have too!! We don't want to see our loved ones and friends worrying about us, day after day, month after month but we have too!! That's not counting all those family and friends who fight their own terrific battle keeping us well, fed, and looked after safe and well.

These last couple of days have been awful for my angel as one night a few days ago was particularly bad as my night terrors and hallucinations showed themselves all night long. The following few nights after, including last night have been all about me waking up screaming and shouting at someone, and Elaine, there as always , arms wrapped around me, rocking me gently until I realise I am only in bed and not stuck in the awful, horrific world I have just left!! I have started to see shadows behind me that make me jump both day and night, and worst of all calling after them as believe me, they are very real to me.

Am I Stressed? NO, in my eyes stress is what you are when out on manoeuvres in minus twenty degree temperatures with a 30lb + pack on and being shot at by the enemy!!

Many people have many different ideas as to why hallucinations and night terrors are prominent along with disturbed sleep when it comes to Lewy body's, including stress (always a favourite of the media), childhood memories, happenings of the last few days and worry. All I can say is I have NEVER witnessed/experienced any of my night terrors or hallucinations whilst awake that would cause me to relive them during the night thankfully. The night terrors are so horrific, graphic and hallucinations so very real to me that sometimes it's so hard to separate reality from my dementia state as I call it.

As time moved on in the early days it was just sporadic during the night but one day, about 2pm in the afternoon I had a full on daytime hallucination. We were sat in a cafe in Barnstaple, it had been a great day and all was well. Elaine asked me what I wanted, tea or coffee and went to the counter to order. Where we sat I could see the lift with people coming and going. I have to admit, I do play a little game of 'Guess the profession' of the people I see when I'm people watching. Do you ever do this? I do like to think I can guess those who are or have been teachers, Dr`s, College professors, Bus drivers, office workers etc. by what they wear and how they look, do you do this? NO? That will just be me then!!!

Then, as I watched the lift doors open for the umpteenth time I sat, rigid to my seat, my breath quickened, my brow started to sweat and my whole body seemed to shake. I watched in horror as the person stepping out of the lift was none other than me!! Yes, that's right, it was me!! Same clothes, same size, same walk, same shoes. A small yelp came from the back of my throat as I tried to shout Elaine. I wanted to turn around and try and find her but my eyes were fixed on this person, ME? Everything went very loud as if someone had turned the volume up on life and I thought at this point I was going to faint. I raised my arm and pointed at him/me and shouted NOOOOO! Elaine must have heard me because she came running over and grabbed the arm I was waving about. "Whatever's the matter she asked!!" I tried to stand, but I couldn't, I was frozen to the spot, mouth open, eyes wide. Eventually I got the words out "LOOK IT'S ME, OVER THERE, walking towards the doors!!! It's me, MYSELF, how can this be Elaine, I asked??" Elaine looked over to where I was pointing and of course didn't see me but someone completely different, just going about his daily business. The next half hour was a mixture of confusion, severe emotions and yes, dare I say embarrassment. Not embarrassment on Elaine's part as she is always the true professional carer and nothing like that fazes her, but embarrassment on my part as I looked at the others in the cafe around me, who met my gaze for a fleeting second then dropped their eyes or pretended they were looking elsewhere. If I am very honest and I would have just witnessed what they had, I would have probably given 'me' the same quizzical look.

The impact of what had just happened was long lasting because no matter how hard Elaine tried to distract me from it and try to help me forget it, it still stays with me to this day!! What I saw, as far as I am concerned, is all very real. It always is to the person experiencing this and it's just as hard for others to believe this is happening as it is for the person going through it. Imagine, just for one minute, sitting in your front room and seeing rabbits, tens of them jumping about right there in front of you. You turn to your family and say LOOK AT THAT!! They all look at you and say LOOK AT WHAT?? No matter how much you try to convince them they are there, they are having none of it and can't see what you see. Would that frighten you? I am sure it would, this is what people with Lewy body's go through on a daily basis. It truly is an awful disease.

June Brown, AKA Dot Cotton, lost her husband to Lewy Body's disease and she coined a phrase that sums up Lewy Body so very well. She says her late husband used to say

'Having Lewy Body's is like having TWO diseases, I HAVE dementia, and I KNOW I have dementia'.

I know exactly what he means. On a very few occasions I remember little bits about what I did the day before. How I screamed, when I saw something that upset me, how I began to run from an unknown, unseen force of evil that was chasing me. The looks and the TUT TUT`S from the general public who don't understand what I am going through. Can you imagine knowing you have done this, and you just know, chances are, you are going to do it again and again? Can you imagine knowing you can sometimes have no control over your actions and how frightening that is? I have to admit, sometimes when this happens, all I want to do is to be put away in a locked room until everybody has forgotten who I am and my actions and illness can cause them no more upset or pain. My illness takes me to some very dark places at times. It empties me of all feeling and leaves me existing from day to day, just muddling through until the depression lifts. Does dementia and depression go hand in hand? In my humble opinion YES, how can it not? How can being told you have something that has no known cure, that takes away your memories of loved ones, friends and acquaintances and removes all dignity not affect you? It has to, you wouldn't be human otherwise. This is why we have to try and get as many as possible to understand the differences between all types of dementia and understand that different behaviours apply.

Do you know one of the most helpful things you can say to someone who tell you they, or a family member or friend has dementia? Ask them "What Type?" yes that's right, "WHAT TYPE?" just those two little words can mean all the difference because it shows you care. It shows you are interested and it also shows you know there is more than just one type. This will mean so much to the person you are talking to and who knows, if they tell you about a type you don't know anything about you might learn something!! Or, it may well be it could be the other way round and you may be able to help them with some of your knowledge. Every now and then within this book I will also insert some of my poems relating to what I have just written, please enjoy…………………

POEM

Oh Dear Sleep!

Oh dear sleep, please come my way,

Pass over me and end my day,

Tormented by my visions past,

Help me slumber, your shadow cast,

Its Lewy Body`s that I fight,

Every second with all my might,

Eyes that see, not always true,

Ears that hear songs so blue,

Laying my head upon my pillow,

O come dear sleep, like a whispering willow,

Take me to a place of hope,

So each day I can cope,

Refresh my mind for tomorrow's day,

To face whatever comes my way

Some people ask me 'does it take you long to write your poetry and verses?' and I have to say once they appear in my mind no not really. Where do they come from? I have no idea and I have often said if my old English teacher Mr Diamond could see me now I'm not quite sure what he would think?

Living with this disease on a day to day basis (please notice I have said living with and not living well, I will explain soon) is so unpredictable but what really gets me sometimes is when they call it a 'JOURNEY'. When they say 'tell us about your JOURNEY with Dementia' JOURNEY? JOURNEy??? For goodness sake, I am not getting on a National coach and having a week in Bognor Regis with it!!

"I AINT ON NO JOURNEY!!!"

I have to live with this disease, day in day out and every long mind numbing minute of it during the night which are always worse. Can we please leave the 'journey' word to the X factor contestants and not relate it to a terminal disease. Could you ever imagine asking someone "Please tell us about your journey with Cancer, or Heart failure? You just wouldn't would you? It wouldn't happen, so why does it with Dementia? I have to say sometimes, some people leave me lost for words, which as you know is very unusual for me, at the way they look at dementia and their attitudes towards it.

In the next chapter I will talk about this and something that's quite controversial at the moment such as living well with dementia or do you say LIVING WELL with or Suffering. Please read on.

But in the meantime, if you do see me jumping, or turning around as though someone has just shouted me, or I look as if I have seen a ghost, give us a smile, a wave and think about this little Lewy Body Soldier just doing his duty!!

The Day I WEPT for the NHS

As I arrived by ambulance at A+E , Torbay hospital, Devon the first thing we noticed were the amount of gurneys lined up with very sick people on them with paramedics, notes in hand, stood by their sides, waiting patiently to be seen. There was no room for another gurney in the aisle so I was ushered from the ambulance and sat on a plastic chair, just taken from the restaurant, as there were no more available anywhere. The only place I could sit was straight, facing the admittance doors which kept opening and closing to the outside elements at a very alarming rate and remembering every time they were opening another poorly person was being admitted.

"Hello, my name is Norrms Mc Namara and I am the founder of the Global Purple Angel Dementia Awareness Campaign, diagnosed myself with Dementia eight years ago aged just 50 yrs old http://www.purpleangel-global.com"

It has been about five years since I was last in hospital and the changes have been a dramatic downward spiral that have even shocked me, and NOT ONE BIT OF THIS is the fault of ANY NHS staff who work there, let's just be very clear on this. As the hours passed and the apologies came thick and fast the first thing I noticed was the sheer look of helplessness and frustration on the faces of the Dr`s, Nurses, Students, Paramedics. Some looked gaunt, some exhausted, but ALL looked on as the endless flow of sick people kept coming in. Cleaners working so hard to keep infections down, volunteers asking if patients were all ok, thankfully I have never been in any kind of conflict zone, but I can only imagine. All this on a normal Monday afternoon, at 3pm, in Torquay.

I was eventually seen and it was explained to me that I would have to have blood tests and an x-ray as I had major breathing problems, coughing fits and a painful lung function. All of which I knew would take to so much time, before being considered for admittance, and whilst all this was going on my 'Angel' Elaine was stood by my side. She had no choice as there were no chairs! The day was broke up a little as because of the Purple Angel Dementia work within Torbay Hospital over the last few years I have met many people, so a few did stop and say hello and wish us well.

After about three hours, (and this was quick), as people had been there over 11 hours, I was told I was going upstairs, out of the melee of A+E and onto what they call Emergency Admittance Ward 4. Now please read this very carefully

When you sit at home and you hear on the news there are no hospital beds, what pops into your mind? All beds are full and you have to wait until a bed becomes available on a ward, right? WRONG!!

As I was wheeled onto E4 Ward, turned into one of the emergency bed bays I had once stayed on before, I saw NOTHING!!

Well, I did, I saw four wing backed chairs where four beds had once been, with three very sick people sat in them with relatives stood around them, and an empty one looking so forlorn in the corner waiting for me. When the NHS say there are NO BEDS, I had no idea they literally meant they have NO BEDS!! I just automatically thought they meant bed spaces!! This is not the case as I know now, and as I sat back and looked around me, it suddenly hit me that our wonderful, beautiful NHS is dying at a very alarming rate and its heart is being ripped away from its very roots and reason she was created. In this one room you could almost hear her cry`s of desperation and longing to go back to the days of when Matrons were feared, yet loved at the same time, where cleanliness was next to Godliness, where straight talking was rife and common sense was king. I was overhearing stories from the other families of how long it had taken them to get this far, and feeling guilty at the same time, knowing I was taking someone else place. Then it happened…………………

A young doctor walked into the room and started to chat to the family next to me. The elderly gentleman who was poorly, and 96 years old I may add, asked the young doctor if they had got their pay rise, this was his very honest answer……………..

"" Thank you Sir, it was never about a pay rise, in fact if I am very honest, I don't want a pay rise, and I am very happy on my salary. I don't do this job because of the money, I do it because I want to help people and help them get well in times of distress. The thing is I am not too keen on doing more hours for less money, that`s all our argument is ""

It was at this I placed my head in my hands and cried. I cried for that young doctor, I cried for every nurse and employee of the NHS in the whole of the UK itself, and I cried for, and with, the NHS Herself, who, even through the depths of despair, still, somehow, manages to function, barely, but function it does and saves the lives of thousands every single day.

Hours later I was taken to a ward called Simpson Ward, and as I passed acute ward after acute ward my spirits were lifted a little as I saw the Purple Angel Dementia Awareness logo standing proudly on each ward entrance doors. As I entered Simpson Ward I tried to smile as I passed the information boards. On the walls of the ward, there was information about Purple Angel Dementia Awareness inside of them.

GOD BESS THE NHS and all who work with her

END OF BLOG   >>>>>>>>>>>>>>>>>>>>>>>>>>>>>>>>>>>>

Chapter Three,

Here we go

Here comes the Controversial bit! (time for a rant)

There has been a lot said lately about the way we word things when it comes to dementia, as well as a lot of reports written and published in the press. I have to say most of it is good advice but there are two things that stick in my throat. The first is when people say 'LIVING WELL' with dementia? Please can someone explain to me how someone can live 'WELL' with such a debilitating disease? How can you 'live well' when the whole essence of your life, memory and life skills are being slowly eroded by a disease that has no cure? Would anybody say you were living well with terminal cancer, or Aids or any other terminal disease?

The term 'living with dementia' in my humble opinion' is much better as it does not give false hope (something the media is infamous for) and tells people you are managing your illness as best you can. Now, here comes the real contentious bit.

Do you say 'Suffering With of from Dementia or not?'

The powers that be say it gives off a negative vibe and doesn't give the disease a true description. Now hang on a minute, I can guarantee there are thousands of carers and family members out there that would disagree!! Let's put it into perspective:

If you are diagnosed with this disease in the early stages, get the right medication and have wonderful support around you, which some of us are lucky enough to have, then by all means please feel comfortable enough to say 'living with dementia' BUT Having watched both my father and grandmother die from this awful disease, having watched their torment, their pain from bed sores, their hunger, thirst and total confusion at not knowing where they were and looking so frightened, there isn't any authority on this EARTH that is going to tell me they were not SUFFERING!!!!

I am also going to be so bold to say when this subject has been discussed on Facebook, 100`s of people agreed. WHO do these people think they are, that they think they can control our lives in such a way, that they can dictate the way we speak, use the English language and restrict our freedom of speech of which we are so famous for here in the UK??

(I told you it was controversial LOL)

But I am not known for holding back and I don't see why I should on this one. This is one subject, as you can tell, that really gets me. It's ok for some of those people in their ivory towers to try and tell us how it should or shouldn't be done, but until you have been diagnosed with this awful disease or you have become a full time carer, both paid and unpaid and experienced the full horrors of it, how can you know??? This is why we should always, at all times, include those living with dementia and their carers in every step, every decision and every policy made. You wouldn't ask a plumber to wallpaper your house would you? So why on earth would you have people making policies, rules and regulations who know nothing or very little about care, instead of asking those in the know. Those troops on the ground that do the care job, day in, day out, 24 hours a day??

Yes we know we are given plenty of 'lip service' and goodness knows there are so many 'tokenistic gestures' of having the odd one or two persons living with dementia on Boards and Committee`s, but the fact is, they are not asking those who have to cope with this, day in day out, and when they do, what are they actually achieving?

One example I can give you was a conference I was invited to in Birmingham a few years ago. I refuse to name who organised the conference as I am not into name calling or petty arguments (life's too short, and it certainly is when you have this disease) but it was all about dementia friendly communities and their progress. As I said it was early days in this concept and a few years ago now. Many attended from all over the UK and it soon became clear that each community was doing things differently, but, and I really do think this is important, I believe it works that way because in each community, each town, each city, the dynamics are so very different and need to be treated as such.

As the day progressed the one thing that became blindingly obvious was the lack of those living with dementia in attendance. So I bided my time and waited for the questions part at the end. When the time for questions was asked my hand shot up and when it was my turn I stood and asked the question I had been burning to ask all day.

I looked around the room and asked "Please, can you all put your hands up in this room if you have a diagnosis of dementia?" I raised mine, and guess what? YEP!! I was the only one in a packed room!! I went on to say "How can you possibly sit here all day and discuss the best way forward when it comes to Dementia friendly communities and not involve those living with dementia?? It went very quiet and the facilitator of the meeting eventually cleared his throat and said "Good question Norrms! This is something we must look at in the future?" Err, horse, door, stable and bolted comes to mind!! Mind you, the box was ticked because they had someone living with dementia at their meeting, ME!!

TOKENISTIC?? YOU BET!

I follow all international conferences etc. where these guys are flying around the globe, slapping each other on the back all discussing how bad things are and how things need to change. But how does that translate down to the person on the street who is chasing a loved one in the middle of the night wearing only pyjamas in the depths of winter? Where do these words and discussions go once the conference is over and how many decisions actually turn into sensible actions which are then applied by Mr Jones or Mrs Smith who have family who have dementia??
I could ask "How much do they cost?" but don't even get me going on that one!! Have you any idea how much these things cost? Room hire, hotel bills, air fare, not to mention food and dare I say drink?? How many memory cafes, day centres or such things could be funded instead of these 'Jolly's' as some call it (not all I hasten to add). In these days of high technology and SKYPE /ZOOM and video conferences surely we could do something different and

plough much needed funds into other, more deserving projects, as well as the important question;
Where does the money come from to pay for all this??

Just a thought?

I can honestly say we have never been abroad to a conference and never would. Yes, we have been asked on more than a dozen occasions but turned them down. This of course is a personal choice and in no way is meant to detract from some of the great work being done around the globe by dementia organisations, but I really do think we should look at how we do things in the future.

I have to say the best conference I was ever asked to attend was in nearby Exeter and was organised by a wonderful friend of mine called Ann Rollings. We worked together in the very early stages of my diagnosis and she has been a hero of mine ever since. I remember her addressing a conference and asking "Do you include people with dementia in all you do?"

When the majority said yes, she looked them all in the eye and said "DO YOU? DO YOU REALLY?? Are they on your steering groups? Your boards? Your decision making teams?? HOW MANY HERE today has brought someone with dementia with them??" I knew then, that day, we would get on and we still do very much. And so to a conference we organised together, but this would be like no other conference that had ever been organised before. This would be a conference that would not only stay in my mind, but with a lot more people for a very long time, WHY? Please read on:

The hotel was booked, table's set, eight of them in all for round table discussions and the Dr`s, Consultants, Hospital staff, nurses etc. were invited along with Carers and people with dementia, but here comes the difference. We were not there to listen to them?? They were there to listen to US!!! YES, that's right, for that day only WE became the facilitators, the carers and the people with dementia not the professionals. They ASKED US what it was like to live with Dementia, and what it was like to be a full time carer, both paid and unpaid!! They sat and listened, open mouthed as we opened our hearts and told them what it was really like, and how hard it was to cope for the carers, loved ones etc. At the end of the conference doors had been opened, minds changed and such a sense of achievement was had by ALL involved.

Has this happened since? To the best of my knowledge Not

as I am aware of. It took one very brave lady Ann Rolling's to organise it and carry it through. I am now hoping someone will read this and replicate that wonderful day, it can be done, we have PROVED it can ....

BLOG   >>>>>>>>>>>>>>>>>>>>>>>>>>>>>>>>>>>>

TORMENTED

BY

CHRISTMAS PAST

AND FEAR OF

CHRISTMAS FUTURE

This time of year is such a confusing time of year, not just for myself, living with dementia, but also for others and their carer`s and loved ones. I try to look back and try to remember what's happened this year. As I start to look into the mirror and take a cold hard look at myself, and this awful illness, the two are now linked forever unfortunately.

I see staring back, a different man from 12 months ago, (I think, it's at this point I look at old photo`s) Is it only me that can see that blankness creeping into my eyes, that disassociation draining from my pupils, or is that just my Illness? Is it ME looking back at ME? Or is it Lewy Body's, smirking behind my smile, laughing at me, tormenting me, taunting me of what's yet to come?

Thoughts come into my mind, happy thoughts, of things achieved, things completed and of things yet to come, until that is, Lewy Body`s walks into the same room in my mind and reminds me of the struggle it has been, the sleepless nights, the hallucinations, the night terrors and the horrors of What Lewy Body`s imposes on my family and I on a daily Basis.

It's at this point the tears start to fall and the feeling of hopelessness envelopes my whole body and mind. As they subside and I wipe away the tears, thoughts turn to next year; well it's only a couple of weeks away. I always like to say, one minute I was watching Space 1999 and the next I was transported into the year 2015, with not that much knowledge of what happened in-between!! And so to next year………………

2016 WOW!! Just saying that sounds so very strange to me, dates, times and months don't come that easily to me these days, but as we all know, time and tide waits for no man or woman, unfortunately, neither does Dementia. If I am very honest, I am dreading the 31st March!! Not the 19th as that's WRAD World Rocks against dementia day, but what about after that? What about when I retire and try to fill my days with other things except the disease that has ruled my life for the last eight years and will end my life if no cure is found?? How do I fill that gap? Most worrying?

Yes of course I am looking forward to spending my time with my 'Angel' Elaine, and yes I am so looking forward to spending more time fishing and gardening, with my kids and going on holiday, but at the end of the day, Lewy Body`s will always be there, chip, chip, chipping away at my family and I. So as you can see, the New Year can be such a confusing time for people like me and their families. So many family members out there must think exactly the same, have the same fears, the same worries, and so many out there with this disease must also think this, even if they cannot speak this.

All that comes to mind at the moment is

DAY BY DAY is all we can hope for, hope this helps

END OF BLOG   >>>>>>>>>>>>>>>>>>>>>>>>>>>>>>>>>>

Chapter Four

Getting a Diagnosis

Poem

WHY ME?

A thousand times this has been asked...

Especially taking my Doctor to task,

What have I done that's so very wrong?

To be punished like this for so long,

Most other illness's come and go,

This one stays as we all know,

It lives within to the bitter end,

Always an enemy, never a friend,

It has no voice, the demon that grows,

Where it comes from no one knows,

It strips you of your very being,

Always there, always seeing,

Causing destruction all around,

Doing all this without a sound,

Taking you away, from your way of life,

Your dignity, children and also your wife,

What is this silent monster I talk about?

What's so quiet with no need to shout?

It's the curse of Dementia, and all it entails,

With its ugly head, it never fails,

To bring such sorrow, upset and pain,

Hiding the sunshine and bringing the rain,

To a life which was once so full,

Always bright and never dull,

But heed my waning bringer of doom,

I promise you this, one day soon,

You will be beaten, over and done,

And out again will come the sun,

I promise this with all my heart,

And once again my life will start,

I will live again, just you wait and see

And never again will you hang over me...

CC Norrms

This could either be the longest chapter you have ever read, or the shortest because of what I am about to say.

You decide……………………..

It is your HUMAN RIGHT to ask for and receive a diagnosis of dementia. Just like it is your human right to be diagnosed with any other disease. There is NO DIFFERENCE< please don't ever forget this. I am asked so many times>

What happens when my doctor says to me 'It's your age' or 'What do you expect at your age?' At this point I would like to ask you a question?

Have you ever walked into a room, stopped, looked around and thought 'I can't remember what I have come in here for???' I would bet a week's wages you are now saying YES! Well, you will be pleased to know, that is Forgetfulness not dementia. We all do that, and sometimes more so when we get a little older, that is certainly not dementia. Dementia is when you sit there with knife and fork in your hands, a meal in front of you and yet you have no idea what to do with the knife and fork. Or it's when you see somebody walking around in their pyjamas outside in the dead of night when it's quite clearly 10c below!! These might seem like drastic ways of putting it, but I think it's the best way to explain what dementia really is. It's not all about forgetting things but about losing your life skills, like not remembering how to tie a tie, fastening your shoelaces, buttoning up your shirt, putting red hot tea or coffee in the fridge, or, in my case, trying to clean my teeth with my razor (there was so much blood!) etc. All these are tell-tale signs. Once again these might seem like extreme examples but all true, so what do you do?

The first thing is to talk about it, ask questions that may seem hurtful but will be so beneficial in the future, questions like (to the person who may have dementia)

How do you feel you are?
Do you feel you're as well as can be?
Is there anything worrying you?

How do you feel about keep forgetting things?

Do you think it's right to walk outside with no shoes on?
And more importantly ....

Do you think it's about time we saw the doctor, just in case? Tell them and reassure them you will be at their side at all times, helping them, listening for them, explaining all to them that they don't understand and you will always be there for them.

Make an appointment

At this point I would like to suggest something that a lot of people don't like doing but I feel is so important you do, which is book a double appointment!! Please insist you want a double appointment which will give you roughly about 20 minutes instead of 10 minutes. WHY? Because when you are sat there and get into full flow, you will need the extra time, I promise you, these things can't be rushed. Depending what the possible outcome is, you will need time to ask questions and reflect on the answers whilst there. Another tip is to write down any questions you may have before you go in, there is nothing worse than coming out of a meeting and thinking I wish I had asked this or that!

You will not, or should not, get a diagnosis there and then. But what you should get is a overview and also a reference to the nearest memory clinic or the Practices CPN (Community Psychiatric nurse) to take what is commonly known as a mini mental test, which consists of about 20 questions, now this where it gets interesting……

Firstly if your doctor doesn't refer you and says it's "just your Age etc" either ……………
Ask for a second or third opinion OR change your GP immediately!! I am not kidding around here; you must be

totally satisfied before you walk away. It really is of the HIGHEST importance that you are. I cannot stress enough how important it is that you get a correct diagnosis because if it is dementia then an early diagnosis can be so important towards living a good life after.

And so to the mini mental test…………………..

Well, back in the day when I was an Alzheimer's society volunteer I was lucky enough to meet many people who worked for the government and also the Department of Health. At one such meeting I brought up the quality of the mini mental test, as I believed then, as I do now, it's seriously flawed. Some of the questions are totally unacceptable and also have no place in today's diagnosis problem. The first major problem is, it's not a standard test all over the UK. It actually differs to where you live in the country and believe it or not, I have heard some doctors don't even use it for fear of being sued by the original people who wrote it, how ridiculous is that??? But wait, it gets even better!! If it's not the same all over the country then how can you produce a clear, accurate amount of statistics of people being diagnosed?? I will not win many friends in the Department of Health by writing this, but hey ho, I am not here to dress it all up for you. I am here to explain how I think, in my humble opinion, where we could

'Do better'.

Then we come to the questions
Q.
Who is the Queen of England??

Err; hang on a minute, dementia is also about short term memory loss and the Queen has been on the throne now for 60years +, Not good.

Q.

Where do you live (what's your address?)

Err; most people who have dementia have lived there for years on end (same as above!!)

Q.

Name three streets near to where you live?

Same as above

and so on,

We know someone who absolutely sailed through the test, got 20 out of 20, came out, sat in the car and his wife asked 'Where have we just been?' He answered 'No idea' and this isn't the first time we have heard this. So, what do you do?

As always it's up to us to convince the doctor or CPN that there is something wrong. How many times have you taken someone to see a doctor and when they are asked "How are you?" they answer "perfectly fine thank you", and for some reason, which only the universe has the answer for, act as normally as you and I and not a trace of dementia can be seen? Sound familiar?? I bet it does!! So, what do we do?

If you are not entirely satisfied with the questions asked during a mini mental test whilst seeking a diagnosis, take a few of your own and ask the doctor, CPN to ask them the questions you have provided, here are some suggestions,

What did you have for your breakfast/lunch/tea?

How did you get here, car/taxi/bus?

What did you watch on television last night?

Where did you go on your last holiday?

And so on, please keep the questions relevant and recent, and don't forget, it's YOUR appointment, your time as well as theirs and you need to make sure you have covered all bases. Depending where you live, unfortunately, will depend on how long it takes and what type of diagnosis you get, this is what I mean. You will either get a diagnosis from the memory clinic or like myself, get a diagnosis from the hospital. My CPN and social worker wasn't happy with my results from the normal tests so I was referred to Torbay hospital for a MRI scan and then a PET scan, this is the difference.

An MRI scan will only tell you what it's not, it's done to make sure there are no brain injuries, aneurisms etc and can come back completely clear. Please don't be fooled, what an MRI scan cannot tell you is if you have signs of dementia or not. This is where the PET scan comes in. The scan I had showed all the brain cells, those which have died and are in the process of dying etc. It showed I had losses in the sides of my brain, back of my brain and some frontal loss, and then a diagnosis of dementia was given. I also asked for a second opinion on this and received the same answer. I still have the paperwork, and probably a good thing too as I know my diagnosis has been questioned a few times by a very small amount of people on social media. Do you know, never once have I thought to question anybody who says they have a diagnosis of dementia, I couldn't, as I know how much of an insult it is to a person who has just been told they have a terminal disease and something there is no cure for, how cruel some people can be??

So, the day came eight or nine years ago when I was called into the consultant's office for my results, and believe it or not his first question was "Do you want to know??" I KID YOU NOT!! I sat there, blinked, decided this wasn't the place to BITE lol, and replied "What do you think I am doing sat here if I didn't want to know? Why would I even be here if I didn't want the results??" He looked perplexed, ignored me and said…………

You have dementia, no doubt about it, my advice is:-
USE IT OR LOSE IT

....
....
....

That was it!! No advice, no follow up appointment, no signposting no nothing!!!! Now, you guys in the medical field, before you get on your high horse, I have stated this was eight or nine years ago and I am the first to admit we have come a long way since then (unless you know different? Answers on a postcard please) we still have a long way to go, but we have come so very far, and this is how I experienced a diagnosis of dementia all those years ago. By sheer luck, my wife, my ANGEL Elaine was a professional carer for over 30+years and she knew where to go, what to do, and what the next steps were we needed to take, but believe me when I say there are so many out there that don't!! They have no idea, and as my great friend Gary le Blanc once put it, 'are left floating in a sea of forgetfulness', the name of just one of his wonderful books.

Some out there have absolutely no idea where to turn, who to see, who to speak to next, and more importantly what about the carer/loved one who has just been told, in a roundabout way, they HAVE to become a full time carer, if not now but in the very near future!! Where do they go, what do they do, and who do they talk to???

I am hoping in the next chapter we can answer some of these questions, so please read on………………..

LEWY BODY`S DEMENTIA,

The Anger within

I can feel it as I sit there, the anger growing and growing inside, nothing has gone wrong, nobody has upset me, and yet I feel so angry inside, so frustrated, so helpless and yet not hapless. I start to tense the muscles in my arms and legs, I squeeze my eyes shut and curl my toes, my fists clench and I squeeze with all my might !!

WHY???

Because I don't know what else to do, Because there is nothing else I can do. I squeeze and squeeze until I shake, it hurts and do it until I can do it no more. My head spins, my eyes hurt and I usually get cramp in my legs and toes. I can do this two, three times a day; I do it more often now than I have ever done. Is it because time is passing me by? Is it because I have no other outlet for my frustration? Or is it because I know deep down I am losing my mind, slowly and agonizingly. The most horrendous thing is, I KNOW this is happening to me!

Some nights are filled with terror, if not night terrors but hallucinations (two totally separate things) which can stay with me for days, sometimes overlapping with the last ones, getting mixed up. Reality merges into a mixture of night and day, screams and shouts and I feel as if I can sometimes live in the here and now, as well as there (wherever there is).

My head feels as if it's about to burst, I can get so very angry within, thankfully not 'without' as yet, and then I sink, I sink oh so slowly into depths of despair. I can feel what I have called my 'concrete overcoat' (depression) slipping over my head and travelling downwards along my arms and towards my feet, whilst all the time, trying so hard to put a public face on as so not to upset my family and friends.

I feel two faced and like a person split in two. Laughing and joking on the outside, yet dying slowly on the inside, with no hope of remission. Why am I telling you all this ?

Because in my heart of hearts, I feel as if I am getting worse. I feel like I am in a desperate race to the finish. Just dementia and I left in the race, side by side, sometimes me winning, sometimes dementia taking the lead. Where is the finish line and how far off? I have no idea, but before I get there I just wanted you all to know;

THIS is the reality of just some parts of my dementia

This is   LEWY BODY`S DEMENTIA

END OF BLOG   >>>>>>>>>>>>>>>>>>>>>>>

Chapter FIVE

WHAT NEXT?????

So as I said , you are sat there, completely perplexed and stunned, if you are very lucky you will know what to do next, but if you don't, what do you do, where do you turn, who do you talk too? All these questions will go through your head very, very quickly. May I respectfully advise you take this next step before you even step out of the surgery/consultants /doctors.

Go straight to the reception desk and make a follow up appointment. Please try and make it within the next two weeks from diagnosis, WHY? because as soon as you walk out of where you are SO MANY questions will begin to form in your minds;

Questions like………………..
What do we do next?
How do we even start to understand what we have just been told?
Can I get a second opinion?

Where do we go for advice?

Will it affect my lifestyle, driving etc.?

Having never claimed benefits in my life, where do I even begin?
Is there any help, I can get and who from?

And the one we all ask HOW LONG??
And many, many more

There will be so many more questions you will want to ask, and NEED to ask, and this is why you HAVE to make a follow up appointment. It doesn't have to be with a Consultant, but can be with a Local CPN (Community Psychiatric Nurse) or someone who works at the nearest memory clinic. I have to say at this point if you have a good and thriving memory café near you, you should be able to walk into one of those and ask for all the advice you need. We offer this at our Purple Angel memory café, and we have a quiet room as well as a social one at the ready so when this happens, we can sit people down and explain as best we can what happens next, and if we don't know the answers, we always know someone who does.

Aren't all memory cafes like this??? I wish they were, but thats not all you can do. Before you have your next meeting please write every question you have down so you don't forget what you want to ask. Please again, as said earlier, it's your time, your life and your future, don't be afraid of keeping them too long as there is nothing worse than coming away and thinking I wish I had asked that!!

Next steps……………..

The best thing to do next is, believe it or not, absolutely nothing. You must take time out to absorb what you have just been told. Take time to go over your questions and hopefully your answers and work out where you go from here. You will be at a huge crossroads of your lives, that I can guarantee, and what you do next will determine, (probably) how the rest of your lives pan out. It will take courage beyond belief and emotion. It will involve lots of tears, but if approached in the right way, it can lead you onto a path that won't be as hard.

Depending what kind of dementia you have will also affect your future. There are so many different types of dementia, over 600 some say, so it's very important when you get a diagnosis to ask which kind, and also ask the difference between the top few. Please remember the word Dementia is just the umbrella term for the many different types, as is for example CANCER. There are many different types of this disease, Cancer of the brain, cancer of the blood etc

Some types of Dementia are:

Alzheimer's
Lewy Body's

Vascular

Frontal lobal

Picks disease (Terry Pratchett died of this unfortunately)

And Korsakoffs Dementia, (caused by Alcohol abuse)

When you are told which one it is, please read up as much as you can about the disease, learn all about it. Google is a wonderful tool for this, but most of all, ask around where you live. The VERY, VERY BEST and MOST reliable information comes from those who are looking after someone with dementia, regardless what the type. These are the family members and carers who are living with or have lived through this. The posh people call them 'Experts by experience'. I call them good honest loving people who didn't ask to become carers but are doing a wonderful job and doing their level best to keep their loved ones safe and give them a better quality of life. These are the people you need to approach, to talk to, to ask anything you want because they have lived, are living, through this and in our experience would be only too happy to help you along. To help ease your pain and share your sorrows because they have been there and know what it feels like.

Incredible people like this come from ALL walks of life, and believe me when I say dementia knows no barriers, has no favour of creed, colour or religion, or most importantly AGE, so why should we? You have to use all at your fingertips. Hopefully by now, one of your questions at your follow up appointment would have been, where do we go now for advice and help? Also, one of the best things to do is to look up local carers groups within your area. Most places have them. Search for memory cafes, there is a directory on the internet that gives you nearly every one that is up and running around the country, where it is, what time it is on and what days.

Here`s the link anyway just in case

http://memorycafes.org.uk/

It's fair to say at this point not all memory cafes are the same and one does certainly not Fit All, a little like dementia friendly communities, but we will come to that a little later in the book. All memory cafes are different, that's a fact. Some are similar, some are not, but what they all SHOULD BE is user friendly. Lately we have been hearing some very worrying reports from some quarters that some memory cafes are actually ASKING as you enter if you have a diagnosis? And if you say no, then you are told you can't come in!! I kid you not!! There aren't enough polite words in the dictionary that explain how bad this practice is and can I just state publically this would NEVER happen at a Purple Angel memory café.

Some are called dementia cafes still, and others have other names, but whatever they are called they all should be non-judgemental and a safe haven for both those with dementia- carers and family members alike. We run ours as it says on the tin, it's a café, you can come and go as you please during the weekly two hours we are open, (on saying that the doors are opened at 1pm for 1.30 and closed around 4pm'ish) we are also open to anyone, even if you have never had a family member with this disease. You are welcome to come and ask advice about it just in case, we will always be there to explain all about it, as I hope other cafes do.

Another way is to quite simply ask friends and neighbours, you will be surprised at how many people either have someone with dementia in their own family, or know someone who has, and have never talked about it. Who knows maybe you could even help them as well as yourself by discussing this and learning as much as you can from each other?

The old saying is 'A problem shared...' Nowadays they say 'it's good to dump your baggage now and again', and believe me, it is!! The trick is knowing where and when, which brings me nicely onto my next subject of WHO TO TELL.

WHO DO I TELL?

This is a very tricky one and really is down to the individual, I will explain what happened to me, our decision and why we did what we did, and then it's up to you my friend`s what you do.

When I was diagnosed I had two choices as I saw it,

1. To tell all

2. To tell nobody

It was as simple as that. So we chose the first option, and this is what happened:

Both my wonderful wife and I sat down and talked about what we should do regarding this, as I said, Elaine had been and still is, a carer for the past 30+ years so. Her first priority was to find out about how I felt about this and explain the obvious and many pitfalls as well as the plusses on choosing which option. The pitfalls, well, there are many. So many people at the time didn't understand what dementia was (a heck of a lot still don't I may add, but we are all getting better at it). There are also plusses as I will explain.

When I told the world I had just been diagnosed with dementia, over 70% of my so called friends on the internet fell away and disappeared into the Ether!! At the time I was not a big internet/computer user so the friends I had made, I cherished as I had known them a while. This came as a massive shock and the feeling of loneliness crept in. I have since come to call this disease 'The loneliest disease of all' and this is one of many reasons why. There was a time which seemed like an age where nobody wanted to discuss this with me, no one seemed to care outside my family (will come to that soon) and my email notifications became less and less. I became very confused and very disillusioned, not forgetting this was a time before they gave me my 'now' medication and I was getting worse by the day, not week, not month, but day; so all things considered it was an awful time for all.

Did I throw my toys out the pram?? Hell yes!! Did I scream and shout "WHY ME?" You bet!! Did I blame my whole family and the rest of the world for this? OF COURSE!!

But as time went on and I got used to the feeling that the whole world wasn't really against me, and not everything was my fault, I began to calm down. I used to think I was right and the whole world was wrong, when actually, it turned out it was me that was wrong and the whole world was right , well, more or less, but I am sure you know what I mean. Eventually things began to pick up a little and I found the more I delved into this disease and its effects on everyday people, then more I felt in control. I started to search for the world Alzheimer's/dementia and so on, I started to look for websites that were specifically made for those with dementia and their carers. Places I could read the real story behind some of the shambolic dressed up versions I had been told about. I wanted to know the REAL TRUTH about dementia and how it was going to affect both my family and myself.

Sadly, even though I found there were a few of these sites available, they all had one thing in common at the time. They were all geared up for carers and family members, and some had no mention whatsoever of those actually LIVING WITH dementia. No special links, no chat rooms just for those with this awful disease, in fact, once again I found I had nowhere to turn.

Things just had to change and change fast! Why were people so convinced that all those diagnosed were too far advanced with this disease that they couldn't converse, couldn't talk to others, and couldn't explain how they felt? Once again another reason why this is such a lonely disease and why it had to change. I am happy to say change it did, not because of me, but because a lot of people seemed to realise this at the same time. It was just one of those times the Universe and Mother Nature did what she does best and give us that little nudge to take things forward. For my part I started to write, and blog on different dementia sites, I started to say HEY, what about those, like myself whom have been diagnosed early? What about those who feel like we have just been thrown on the scrap heap with nowhere to turn, and more importantly, what about OUR VOICES!! Why cannot they be heard like anybody else's??

I have to admit, in the most, I got pleasant and courteous replies, but some I got were of total disbelief, and indeed one site which I won't mention actually blocked me because they could not believe I could write and still have dementia!! All this made me even more determined to have my say, all this made me dig my heels in and want to tell the world I was still here, living breathing and living my life as best I could despite what life had thrown at me, and as most of you know, that's exactly what I did.

I have to say, at the time of writing this, I now have over 4,800 friends on Facebook. Over 2,500 on Twitter, I run a page called Dementia Aware on Facebook which has over 18,500 current member`s from ALL over the world, that's members, not likes,

Link is

https://www.facebook.com/groups/250325295027020/

and a few other dementia related pages and blogs with 1,000s of others who read and help each other. I also, as most of you know, head up the Global Purple Angel Dementia Awareness Campaign, which is now established in 38 countries at this time of writing and have over 530 Purple Angel ambassador's worldwide, and guess what?

EACH AND EVERY ONE of them knows I have dementia and DON'T CARE that I do!!!!

So to all those who turned away and left me I do not blame you if you were frightened and didn't understand the disease, I always say 'You don't know what you don't know until somebody teaches you'

To the others?? Well, I will let you guess the answer to that one!!

So in conclusion, I and my family decided to tell the world I had dementia. It wasn't as easy as you have just read and may not be what you want to do, that's your choice, all I can say is it worked for us. We got through the bad times and now things have levelled out to a certain degree. What I will say is, when it comes to telling children go ahead, why, because they get it!! They will understand it is just a disease of the brain, they KNOW you can't catch it, they know it's not airborne or contagious, and remember, these children are the future and they will reduce the stigma of this awful disease as they grow up, which will make things even better for all

BLOG   >>>>>>>>>>>>>>>>>>>>>>>>>>>>>>>>>>>>

DO THOSE WITH DEMENTIA REALLY CHANGE THAT MUCH??

Do people who have dementia change? YES!!

BUT Do they REALLY CHANGE THAT MUCH ????

This is a question I have been asking myself for a while now. I myself, as you know was diagnosed with dementia eight years ago, and lately wrote the poem 'I JUST WANT TO BE ME AGAIN' (at the bottom of this post)

But I have many questions about this. We know that in the main, dementia is a short term memory loss disease and in the latter stages they find it hard to remember names and faces of the closest of family members. But if we remember to keep the 'SHORT TERM' memory loss part of it, this only encompasses a small part of their life. An example is they cannot remember what they recently had for supper, or what they may have done yesterday, the day before or even ten years before, but if they are 80 years old, that is only a small part of their life. They can't remember recent events, but have so many memories of many years they can remember. !!

They have so much to discuss, so much to talk about and so much to do. As you know, at the Global Purple Angel Dementia Awareness Campaign is 'INCLUSION AND ENGAGEMENT AT ALL TIMES' and when this is upheld, when communicating with those with dementia, there is an absolute wealth of experience we can listen to, share and sit absolutely amazed at what they tell us; which, as an added bonus, can be shared with our children and grandchildren so they themselves can see far past the illness and see the person they were before dementia came along.

'MEMORIES ARE THERE TO BE SHARED'

Yes, it's great to share memories, but what about the physical side of it?? Now I don't mean anything too much for obvious reasons, but in care homes there are many people who are prone to wandering, or those that have just got into that routine of coming down, sitting and looking at four walls, when there are so many other things that they can do!!

INCLUSION means just that!! It's not all about sitting there chatting to them all day. Goodness knows the care staff are busy enough and even though I am sure lots would love to do this, I just know they are so busy and understaffed that sometimes this is not possible. But what about asking them to do what they used to do? What about asking them to help tidying the magazine rack, the bookshelves, maybe even a little polishing, and dusting? How about suggesting helping (with supervision) in the kitchen?? Just because they have dementia doesn't mean they can't beat an egg, dry a plate, or mix a bowl of flour?? This applies to both sexes and there are plenty, including myself, who loved to cook!!

Gardening, ok, I mean seeding and potting on, maybe a little raking and tidying up, but the POINT is they are active again, they are doing things they have ALWAYS done, and just because they have lost a few years of memories doesn't mean they have become completely immobile, and in some cases, can't remember what they did in their youth!

As a person with this awful disease, my advice would be please don't wrap those up in cotton wool that do not need it and let them live their lives to the very best of their ability.

I hope this helps, please share, and thank you ALL for EVERYTHING you do

Norrms and family

xxxxxxxxxxxxxxx

POEM

I JUST WANT TO BE ME AGAIN!!

I am me !!

I am sure I am me !!

What is, or who is the real me ??

Will I ever be the same me again ??

I can't be the same me I used to be!!

I am he who is now, not then!!

So who is me ??

So confusing !!!

Am I defined by my dementia?

Or does my dementia define who I am?

So many unanswered questions

Who will be the future me?

So, this is me now, is it?

Is this who I want to be?

But who do I want to be ?

I JUST WANT TO BE ME !!!!

END OF BLOG   >>>>>>>>>>>>>>>>>>>>>>>>>>>

Chapter Six

Taking the next steps

So by now you should know what kind of dementia it is. You know the symptoms? Hopefully you are getting the right medication, and getting some sort of help, right??

Probably wrong I'd bet, and here`s WHY??

Because many of us believe that there are plans in place for these kind of things, after all there is with any other type of disease, so why not dementia? Why not indeed!! Unfortunately it's not like that in REAL LIFE, and in the next few minutes or so I hope to give you some home truths, some of which will astound you, some will disturb you and some will downright shock you! But they are true to the best of my knowledge and I hope to also tell you how you can do things a little differently and get the help you will so desperately need. Always remember you CANNOT do this alone, as much as some of we think we can, and as much as things have changed up this year of 2016, it's certainly not something that is automatically given to you. You have to go out and fight for these things and this help, so here goes…………………..

Will someone come and knock at your door and offer help?
NO

Will someone come round and offer to sort out your benefits unless you ask them to?
NO

Will your doctor automatically refer you to a CPN and social worker straight away to get you respite help?
No

You're probably sat there thinking "You're not helping Norrms"

But I hope I am, as I am telling it as it is. Elaine had to go out and FIGHT for everything we have. Benefits, care package, direct payments, (a must if you live in the UK), and so much more. There is so much help out there, carers meetings, therapy (often for free) counselling, befrienders, helpful apps that can help with daily tasks, dementia friendly places, memory cafes. I could go on and on, but you have to go out and search for these things. Elaine and I once worked with the Department of Health on a website which put all of these services in one place on the computer, only to be told two years later and after a lot of hard work that there was no funding available for it??

Contact your local Alzheimer's society or Purple Angel Ambassador. There is also Dementia UK, Admiral Nurses (I will talk about them soon), Lewy Body's Association,

Vascular and Frontal Lobal groups on Google and Facebook, if you are computer literate, and if you are there are so many forums you can contact. Carers UK is also another one you can chat with other carers, all these numbers and address will be at the back of this book to help you.

The road in front of you will be a long one but doesn't have to be a lonely one. Take your time, sit back and prioritise. Make a plan and implement that plan bit by bit, you can't do it all at once. What or who comes first, the person with dementia or your own wellbeing? Who looks after the person with dementia if you the carer/caregiver are ill? All these things need to be sat down, talked about and a plan put in place. I think depending on what stage the person with dementia is, will be dependent on how you prioritise, it's up to you, it's a personal thing, but either way a plan needs to be put in place.

The next subject is another that needs to be discussed but is certainly a lot harder than forming a plan. It involves End of Life care. Some very hard questions, probably lots of tears and a subject no one likes to talk about which is death and after death, but all this comes under the same heading and if you allow me to, I will explain how Elaine and I approached it;

I was first diagnosed with heart failure fourteen years ago so five or six years before my diagnosis of dementia. We had our wills put into place and all was covered, well, that is before dementia came along! We now realised this was a whole new ball game and we had to change the goalpost, so to speak. The first thing we did was to take the phone off the hook, make a coffee and sit at the dining table (optional LOL).

We knew it was going to be a long night but we also knew it was something we had to talk about, openly and honestly. Once again the question was asked how long? Once again it was a question neither of us could answer so we decided together that the next 15 years needed to be spoken about.

Firstly Elaine explained the difference between Power of Attorney and LASTING Power of attorney, a HUGE difference depending which country you are in (we are in the UK) and the easiest way I can think of explaining this is always go for LASTING power of attorney so you have all the say, ALL OF THE TIME. It's really as simple as that and the doctors and consultant's cannot take these decisions out of your hands.

That decision made it was onto the next question. What goes into it, where do I want to end up, what kind of care do I want, how do I want the burial to go, who attends, who doesn't (LOL) what music, hymns etc. All these things need to be discussed and written down. I have to admit it was at this point I broke, and I broke down spectacularly. Everything seemed so final, so desperate, I felt as if time was running out and I didn't have that long left, 15 years, 15 years repeated itself in my head, such little time seemed to have passed since I was 21 let alone 15 years into the future!! We held onto each other as if we were the only people in the world, and for that particular time we were. We have never felt as close as we did that night, but deep down we knew we were doing the right thing, and here's why.

When someone asks how long have you and Elaine been together I always answer "FOREVER". Not that's a bad thing, in fact quite the opposite, I feel I have known her all my life and it's MY honour to do so. So why, when It comes to organising things like the funeral, hymns etc would I be so selfish as to leave it all to her? Why would I think 'It won't affect me, I won't be here'. How could anybody do that? How can you leave a loved one thinking "Did I do the right thing? Is it what they would have wanted? Did I pick the right hymns, give them the best send-off I could?"

There is no getting away from it was a very long night, with even more tears and tantrums, from me, not Elaine I might add, but once done, it was done. The following day I knew we had done the right thing because Elaine said she felt so much better and felt as if a weight had been lifted off her shoulders. You have to share the responsibility and get your house in order as they say, and whilst well enough, this can be done.

Once again this chapter is all about helping yourself to make your life a little easier after diagnosis. Yes it can be such hard work at times, but the point is, once the path forward is prepared it can be a little easier, as someone once said (not me by the way);

If you fail to prepare,
Then you might as well prepare to fail

Something I have tried to live by all my life.

DEMENTIA HAS MANY FACES

So, there we stood in the kitchen, chatting about the day, we had just visited Berry Pomeroy Castle cafe and tea rooms, the scones just LITERALLY melt in your mouth, highly recommended, when the door to the front room opened and in strode the angriest man I had ever seen !!! I JUMPED in front of Elaine and shouted WHO ARE YOU?? GET OUT GET OUT!! HOW DARE YOU!! Just then he lunged at me, but I reacted first and went straight towards him!! At the same time Elaine had wrapped her arms around me as best she could and with a HUGE effort pulled me back screaming "ITS NOT REAL,ITS NOT REAL" Just for a moment time stood still, we were both frozen in the moment. Elaine , myself, and the very Angry man suspended in a timeless animation for a split second, and then he was gone. One minute there, the next not. All I could do was stand there in the arms of Elaine, shaking with both fear and anger.

When people say to me 'You don't look like you have dementia?' they don't see this side of it. When people say 'you look really well', its lovely to hear, but, thankfully, they don't realise that this can happen at any time, day or night, this was 3.30pm in the afternoon, and when some say you look drained and tired, THIS IS WHY !!

This disease is truly awful, someone said last week that I do not represent the true face of dementia, and do you know something I agree with him 100%!!! Why, because DEMENTIA has so many, many faces, and I am just but one of them.

END OF BLOG   >>>>>>>>>>>>>>>>>>>>>>>>>>>>>>>>>>>>

Chapter Seven

The Birth Of The Purple Angel

In my last books its written and been well documented
what happened when I walked into a Torquay shop and
how the TDAA (Torbay Dementia Action Alliance) was born,
but what about the Purple Angel Campaign? How did that
come about and how did we get so big so fast? Hopefully in
the next few pages/chapters all will become clear. Though I
have to admit, I still have problems understanding how we
have managed to come so far in such a short time.

If anybody is expecting the next bit of the book to be about
deriding other dementia organisations they couldn't be
more wrong!! Much has been said about the Alzheimer's
society and ourselves, and not much of it good or
productive. All I will say is my hope has always been, and
will always be, we can work together to improve the lives of
others. We are on the same side really and want the same
thing; we just do things differently, but want the same
ending. At a conference recently I was asked why the Purple
Angel and forget me not badges could not become as one as
it's all a bit confusing, I answered in this way.

In sport, football in particular, we have the Premiership and all the different football leagues, we all play the same game, want the same goals (pardon the pun LOL) and want to do our best. Yet the teams all wear different strips, have different badges, we all support different colours and there's no confusion there, we all know what an Arsenal shirt looks like, a Celtic shirt, or a Manchester City shirt looks like and can resonate with that, so why should there be a difference? We have different companies all over the UK manufacturing the same goods and all you have to do is a little research and choose the one you want. It really is no different. Yes, in a perfect world we would all work together and everything would be hunky dory, but how boring would it be if we all supported the same team??

The person who asked me this was quite happy with the answer as I hope you are. Will we, (the Purple Angel) ever sit across a table with the Alzheimer's society and discuss how we can take things forward TOGETHER ?? I certainly hope so and our door is forever open, now, that bit is over its time to move on and tell you all about how the Purple Angel was created.

The Torbay Dementia Action Alliance was formed about four years before the Purple Angel. The TDAA had no logo and one day it was suggested that we have one!! So, I asked on Facebook if someone would draw the TDAA a logo that would fit perfectly with what we were doing around Devon (little did I know at the time what would happen!!) I have to admit I was sent some wonderful images, some even in 3D, you really are a clever lot out there. Then, my good friend and now Co-Founder of Purple Angel, Jane Moore, showed me a doodle she had drawn on what I could only describe as a Crumpled piece of paper!!

On it was drawn a very rough outline of what was quite clearly an angel and coloured purple. When I asked what it was, this is what she said, "In every book you have written, you have always called your lovely wife 'Your Angel'. So that's where that comes from. I have coloured it purple as it's a healing colour, and HEY PRESTO!! The Purple Angel was BORN!!!

The logo was printed on all the volunteers Tee shirts who helped out at the TDAA events, and that was that! Or so we thought????

Shortly after announcing to the world that this was the new logo of the Torbay Dementia Action Alliance the most incredible thing happened. The WHOLE WORLD and HIS WIFE wanted to know what the logo was and what it meant?? Some thought there was a religious reason behind it, no, certainly never crossed our minds. Some thought it was a cult of some sort (I kid you not, and have heard worse since LOL) But what did happen was so many people across the world fell in love with this simple but effective logo that it soon became apparent the Torbay Dementia Action Alliance should not keep it as their own logo, that would be so selfish. So the decision was made by Jane Moore, myself and the steering group of the TDAA we should share it with the world, with no fear or favour. That it should be FREE for all to use under the banner of raising awareness of dementia, providing it always stayed a non for profit symbol.

Well, within three months Jane and I lost count of the amount of people wanting to use this logo worldwide. Someone once asked me why I thought it had become so successful so quickly and this was my answer;

Quite simply put, The dementia organisations worldwide all have their own logos, the Alzheimer's Society UK, Dementia UK, Brace UK, Alzheimer's association USA, Alzheimer's Australia and so on. Indeed the International organisation Alzheimer's International has its own logo, but what the world didn't have was a WORLD LOGO for every type of dementia!! We wanted to encapsulate ALL types of dementia and make sure NOBODY slipped through the net, and that's exactly what happened. As you know, at this time of writing this, we are now established in 38 Countries around the world and COUNTING. We also, at this moment have over 530 PA Ambassadors (and counting) globally who have their own teams of people. We have memory cafes worldwide; we even have Purple Angel Cities thanks to my wonderful friend Kathy Broggy in the USA. We also have, thanks to one of the hardest working PA ambassadors in the world Gary LeBlanc, now have hospital wristbands with a Purple Angel printed on it for those with a diagnosis and admitted to hospital in many areas of the USA, a world first!! This is just a small glimpse of what we have done since we SHARED the purple Angel logo with the world. But how did the OFFICIAL PURPLE ANGEL campaign start??

READ ON ……………………………

One night, about three years ago, Elaine and I were sat at home watching the local news, we were both in tears as they had just reported that a lady had been missing from nearby Exeter and they had found her dead, she had dementia. I felt as if I had lost one of my own and Elaine, a professional carer for over 30 years + was devastated. I just sat there shaking my head and thinking there just HAS to be something we can do in this day and age surely. The next thing on the TV was something about GPS systems and all of a sudden the idea came to me. It wasn't a new idea and certainly wasn't mine, because as I Googled GPS and dementia there were some devices already out there, but the idea was born to hold a fundraiser, make as much as we could, buy as many of these devices and GIVE them to those in need, especially in and around Torbay. Again little did we know what was waiting around the corner.

About this time we were in talks with a company from London called Ostrich UK who loved what we were doing around Torbay, loved our simple way of doing things, our honesty and vision. They wanted to help us further our awareness campaign and offered, FOR FREE, to redesign and print posters for us along with other materiel. What a Godsend it was. Up to this point we were going around handing out photocopies of what we had written to help shops etc, now we had glossy, professional posters for all to keep and they have been used ever since. When I met the CEO of Ostrich UK, Laurence Kelly, I just happened to mention (as you do) our upcoming charity event to raise funds to buy GP's for those with dementia, and after a very short conversation the idea was born to actually produce our own, with no cost at all to the TDAA or Purple Angel. (Ostrich care we will always be forever grateful for this).

These would be produced with the electronic know how of Ostrich UK and also the uppermost input from myself, a person living with dementia, Elaine, a carer, the police, the NHS and other bodies. Within months our dream came true and "BOB" GPD for those with dementia as its known became a reality and is now available WORLDWIDE

Website http://www.bobtechnology.co.uk/

And now onto the Fundraising night, I have always said the people of Torbay are some of the most generous people I have ever met. We needed a venue for the night and the incredible people who own Babbacombe Theatre let us have full run of the place, for one night only completely free!! (Normally £800 to rent) We also needed a big name and they don't come any bigger than the Plymouth Military wives and tenor Tyrone Piper Power, who also gave their services for free, along with genius musical producer Rob Young, and so the scene was set.

That night we raised in excess of £5,000, that night we knew we could afford to BUY many with dementia a GPS to keep them safe, JOB DONE ?? Not quite……………………..

Shortly after, and after many, many, many weeks of negotiation we are so proud to announce the HUB, the Call centre for the new BOB GP's for the whole of the UK and beyond was to be based right here in Torquay, a proud day indeed!!!

Then one wonderful glorious day in November did we award Purple Angel ambassadorship status to no less than 50 people from across the world, this was the invite………………

INVITATION to Ostrich Purple Angel Ambassadors

You are invited to attend the inaugural ceremony where you will be officially appointed and welcomed by Norman McNamara and the Ostrich team who support his work

On

16th November 2013 from 14.00-16.00

At

The Palace Hotel

Esplanade Road, Paignton, Devon TQ4 6BJ UK

Light refreshments will be served after the ceremony

Please RSVP

What an incredible day that was. People came from all over the UK, and the world to join the Purple Angel campaign. Little did we know, nearly three years on, it would turn into the global phenomenon it is today, and so proud to say it's still running now with the same values as when we started. Not for profit, no one ever takes a wage and we are all volunteers. I like to think of it as the

LARGEST COMMUNITY GROUP in the WORLD

And still we grow ……………………………..

BLOG   >>>>>>>>>>>>>>>>>>>>>>>>>>>>>>>>>>>>>>

BEFORE MY DEMENTIA, why haven't you asked??

My Name is Norrms, and I have dementia, but before I had dementia, do you know who I was or what I have done?? If not, why not??

When I left school my first job was as a painter and decorator but I was scared of heights so that didn't last long!!

I applied for the RAF but was turned down because of childhood heart problems

I worked in Cordon Bleu, Asda, and the Cotton Mill as a Mule Piecer (this is when I was made to grow up, though some still say I haven't yet ha ha!)

I drove a four and a half ton Lansing Bagnall fork lift truck for years in the good inwards department of automotive products.

I once woke up in a bedsit after being made redundant and was so fed up of being out of work and broke, I packed a knapsack, a tent and a few things on a Tuesday morning and hitchhiked it to Dover, there I caught a ferry to France, 72 hours later I was in Bordeaux, on my own, and lived there for a year!! I picked cherries, grapes and worked in the kitchen of various restaurants.

I came back and there was still no work so I went to live in Dublin and Country Clare for a year to work on farms and in pubs.

Back on English soil, after meeting my Angel Elaine, I did various temping jobs, as this always paid a few bills and put bread on the table as they say, this included the wonderful jobs of packing frozen burger buns, packing pens in pencil cases, sorting out soiled sheets from the operating theatres in our local hospital, and even spending seven days sat on a box in a warehouse cutting down the whiskers of Lion King toys because EU rules stated they were too long!! I KID YOU NOT!! Ha Ha.

I've worked in a paint factory, a paper mill, came down to Devon and filled shelves, collected hotel laundry before finally working at Focus Do It All and becoming a manager, something I am very proud of even today as I come from very humble beginnings and poor education.

My point is my friends, Dementia has only played a very small part in my life, as it does in anybody's life, but the lives led before are wondrous!!! Exciting!! Sometimes dangerous!! And sometimes downright SILLY!! But yet they have been lived!! These are not just stories that need to be told, but also need to be listened to and remembered!!

Please all, the next time you speak and sit with somebody who has this awful disease, ASK them what it was like growing up, and I can assure you, no matter how well you think you know them, they will always be able to tell you that little something you didn't know before!!!

Much love, Norrms Mc Namara

Diagnosed with dementia aged 50, now aged 58

END OF BLOG

>>

Chapter Eight

Time for a bit of poetry

Hi, I am asked so many times if I ever publish the poems I write about living with dementia. I have in the past (details at the back of the book) written three books about my fight with dementia, one of them is a dedicated poems book. I always thought it was a little unfair to write a poetry book and a normal book about living with this disease when I could incorporate both for the same price more or less. So that's what I did with my last book 'Silent Voices' and will do with this one, so here goes, a few poems from the heart, trying to explain a few of my on-going struggles, but also my hopes for the future, as I truly believe I do have one ....

A FLEETING GLIMPSE

My heart is breaking piece by piece

From dementia's clutches, I want release,

My body aches, my eyes they weep

As ever closer to death I creep

Forever falling into a deep abyss,

Screaming out for one last kiss,

From lips that are oh so true,

My darling Angel, I love you,

Friends and families, images bare,

A fleeting glimpse of those who care,

For Life itself is but a glance,

A hurried breath, a quickened dance,

A dance that will not last forever,

Because dementia`s far too clever,

So make the most, one and all,

Before Dementia comes to call.

BEHIND THE SMILE

Behind the smiles lies a broken man,

Shattered in so many pieces,

Just wanting his old life back again,

Away from Dementia`s crease`s,

Behind the smile, the man cries out,

To all who want to hear,

But his sobs and woes are deafened out,

By the sound of drying tears

Behind the smile, is a man so scared?

Shaking every day,

From fears and tribulations,

That often comes his way,

Behind the smile, the man's worn out,

So tired from lack of sleep,

Secretly waiting for the end,

To death he slowly creeps,

But behind the smile, of this broken man,

Lays the person he once was,

Still smiling to one and all,

WHY? Well just because!!

My Dementia, ITS NOT MY FAULT!

Please remember, when I forget your name,

It's Not My Fault!

Please remember when I call you by someone else`s name
It's Not My Fault!

When I have little accidents

It's Not My Fault!

When I stare blankly, upwards and cannot understand what
you're saying

It's Not My fault!

Please remember when I spill my tea down my front

It's Not My Fault!

When we visit family and I cannot remember the children`s
names

It's Not My fault!

When I look so sad I could cry (and quite often do, in
private)

It's Not My Fault!

When I scream with frustration because I can't say the
words I want to

It's Not My Fault!

When I disappear into a world of my own for hours

It's Not My Fault!

Please remember if I fall or step out in front of traffic

It's Not My Fault!

BUT MOST OF ALL PLEASE REMEMBER

If forget to say goodbye, or "I LOVE YOU" right at the END?

It`s Not My Fault, But DEMENTIA`S FAULT

I only wish it was, it would make life so much simpler

....

DEMENTIA`S FURY

As darkness closes all around,

From the cold dark night, not a sound,

Then suddenly, from deep within,

A muffled cry, before troubles begin.

Rising from the depths below,

Dementia`s anger begins to grow,

Flooding your mind with angst and screams,

Showing itself as horrendous dreams.

You try to wake with no avail,

A quiet night has just set sail,

Instead arrives dementia's fury,

Sole executioner, without a jury.

Tormented soul`s appear to sneer,

Taunting you with their fear,

The volume builds within your head,

Filling you with immediate dread.

Inside your sleep, it's not so kind,

Twisted shapes within your mind,

YOU SCREAM !!!! with arms and legs amiss,

For peaceful sleep, a rested bliss.

Eyes open wide as you look around,

Searching, straining, for that awful sound,

As Dementia`s Fury fades away,

For me it's just another day.

WITHIN THE DARKNESS OF MY MIND

Within darkness of my mind, feeling so alone,

Trying to make sense of it, shivering to the bone,

It's been 7 long years since dementia came, affecting all I do,

Slowly erasing the memories I have, life style actions too.

I remember the day so very well, the doctor said to me,

'Dear sir you have Dementia, that is plain to see',

The scan has shown your brain cells, are slowly dying one by one,

It was at this point, I was sure, my life was all but done.

But then the fight within me, raised its voice on high,

It shouted "DO YOUR BEST DEMENTIA" I'm not prepared to die!!,

Since that day, we have walked tall, and fight each and every day,

Praying that Dementia, never comes your way.

WALKING INTO WINTER

Walking into winter, with dementia at my side,

Is not something I would wish, and yet I must abide,

Some days are full of sorrow, with a very heavy heart,

Yet others bright and breezy, just like a brand new start.

Every day is different, never knowing when

Dementia's demons visit, time and time again,

Sometimes it drains my soul, my life force ebbs and flows,

There are times I do admit, I feel like letting go.

Then I look around, and see the smiles that come my way,

It is then I know, my fight will always stay,

So COME ON dementia`s demons, fight me IF YOU DARE!!

You will never win, please everybody SHARE !!!!

PLEASE DONT PITY ME

Please don't pity me because I have dementia

What do you see when you look into my eyes?

Do you see a blank stare, a sorrowful face?

And yet? You don't see what I see........................

I see my childhood friends, playing abundantly

I see my wonderful mum and Dad guiding me in life

My brothers and sisters are still young as we play in the garden

The town where I was born hasn't changed a bit

The school still stands were I went

On the park we spent so many hours on, the gates are still open

I can still smell the forest we played in

The food tastes just the same as it did,

And the sun is still as hot.................

Please don't pity me because I have dementia

Just because I am regressing isn't such a bad thing,

Where I am now, I have no worries, no bills, no expenses,

Where I am now is a happy place,

I am sorry if I don't remember you as who you are,

But if I remember you as my sister, or mum,

That is a huge compliment, so please don't be sad,

Be happy for me, after all.......................

I am getting a Second chance at visiting my CHILDHOOD

HOW MANY CAN SAY THAT???

<u>YOU SEE ME, AND YET, YOU DON'T KNOW ME?</u>

You see me, and yet you don't know me?

You hear me, and yet you ignore me?

You talk about me, and yet, don`t talk to me?

You laugh at me, yet I am not funny?

You Pity me, and yet know nothing about me?

You whisper about me, and yet I can hear you!

You dress me, and yet never ask me?

You feed me, and yet I don't feel hungry,

You wake me, and yet I am so tired,

You speak at me, and not too me?

And yet I am still me, I was me before my dementia, and I will still be me at the end, so why, I ask again

YOU SEE ME AND YET YOU DON'T KNOW ME?

WHEN TIME STANDS STILL

When all around you stop and stare,

When it feels as if nobody cares,

You want to scream, but you don't dare,

Dementia`s mist drags you afar,

When Time Stands Still.

When you look but cannot see,

You can't quite believe, what will be,

You begin to shout "Dear God WHY ME?"

All you want, is to be dementia free,

When Time Stands Still

When you awake, and feel so alone,

Family and friends surround, yet feel on your own,

No one to talk to, no one to phone,

Nightfall arrives and you're chilled to the bone,

When Time Stands Still

As you pray for that elusive cure,

Each day passes you're not so sure,

Dementias fingers continue to lure,

And they wrap around one`s so pure,

 When Time Stands Still

 You take small steps day by day,

On tear stained pillow your head will lay,

All your demons, you want to keep at bay,

To be forever free of dementia`s way,

THIS is when time STANDS STILL

TEARS OF A CLOWN

Tracks of tears down a reddened face,

Tears that fall in a similar place,

Eyes that stare through a curtain of lace,

Are these the tears of a clown?

A smile that could light up the sky,

Hidden behind an all familiar sigh,

From deep inside an inhumane cry,

Are these the tears of a clown?

Convincing many that all is well,

A story, far too horrid to tell,

Wanting release from this living HELL

Are these the tears of a clown?

Dementia invades my every act,

The two together, in a Devils Pact,

But I won't give in, and that's a fact!!

Are these the tears of a clown?

DEMENTIAS GATE

The Night Terrors come thick and fast

And always with an unfamiliar cast,

People's faces come and go,

Screaming obscenities high and low,

Doing their best to do me harm,

Dragging me, from dear sleeps calm,

I awake, not knowing where I am,

Trying to make sense, if I can,

But all my demons are still there,

Spitting, swearing, they don't care,

With both arms flying all around,

Trying to defeat the moving ground,

That flies up into my face,

With evil intent, and at such pace,

Eyes blood red, full of hate,

Looking at me, is Dementia`s Gate,

Trying to drag me from all I know,

Into despair, far below,

But just as I feel myself falling,

A familiar voice is gently calling,

It's ok Norrms, it's just your dementia,

And brings me back from this latest venture,

I sit there, sweating and shaking,

From something which is not of my making,

My 'Angel' Elaine`s arms surround me

Keeping me safe from what may be,

Another night has come and gone,

At the rising of the sun,

But what of tonight, what will be?

We will just have to wait and see.

LEFT OUT IN THE COLD

Do you remember Christmas past?

Where older memories seem to last,

Far gone times, and days of old,

When winters were, oh so cold,

The snow it drifted, high and low,

Blown along like seeds that sow,

But what of last year, or the year before,

Not one memory comes through the door,

Of my mind, while dementia`s here,

Robbing me and feeding my fear,

Older memories are all well and good

And remembering them, we all should,

But just for once, it would be nice,

To check the calendar and throw the dice,

And have a memory of just last week,

This is not too much to seek,

Memories of a film, a face or a meal,

Any one of these would mean a great deal,

No matter how hard I try,

None of these memories come fluttering by

So here I sit, with memories of old,

Cast adrift, out in the cold.

This Is How Life Is

Summers Come, Summers Go,

Autumn falls, Winter snow,

Spring arrives and flowers grow,

This is how life is

As we grow, eyes are wide,

Taking in all with pride,

Family and friends by your side,

This is how life is,

Middle age comes to all,

Expectations begin to fall,

Then old age comes to call,

This is how life is

Feeling tired, looking back,

Remembering little, losing track,

Ever smaller the family pack,

This is how life is

Dementia calls, so alone,

In your mind, you're all own,

Oh how I wish, someone would phone,

This is how life is

Does Dementia win? Well, that depends,

At last!! Surrounded by your friends,

Your love for life will NEVER END,

This is how life is

IN CASE I FORGET

In case I forget when glancing at you,

The one who makes me complete,

Alzheimer's may have won with my mind,

But my heart it will never defeat,

In case I forget the children we`ve raised,

Or the hundreds of stories I've told,

Shed not a tear for blessed are we,

Who forget one day we are old,

In case I forget to tell you how much,

You're cherished and treasured each day,

My best friend beside me to brighten the path,

And carry me all of the way,

I may greet you someday, with questioning eyes,

As a stranger with whom I've just met,

Still, I love you my darling, with all of my heart,

Remember...... In case I forget

ECHOS

Echos of the years gone past,

Fleeting memories that never last,

Weathered face, weeping eyes,

Confused state, anguished cries

Where did all the good times go?

Now lost forever, in the flow,

The tidal flow that is Dementia,

All hope lost, with no new ventures,

Until that day, that glorious day,

When we hear, someone say,

A CURE IS FOUND, all is well,

No more to suffer, this Dementia Hell,

And once again the world will sleep,

A peaceful life, Is ours to keep.

SIX YEARS GONE

Six years gone and still no cure,

So much love from one so pure,

My Angel waits within the wings,

Beating heart that used to sing,

Now falls silent, patiently so,

Waiting, willing the world to show,

We Have a Cure! All Is Well!

Time to END this Dementia hell,

Tears will flow on this day,

Tears of happiness may I say,

My Angel Elaine will turn to me,

To say "The Futures ours to see"

The world will sigh, with relief,

As we say goodbye to this Dementia thief

PLEASE

Please give me a smile:

It will mean so much:

Come on, give us a wave:

And watch my eyes wave back

Ask how I am:

Its shows you care:

Ask how I've been:

I promise I won't tell you the truth:

Tell me a Good Joke:

I promise I am laughing on the inside:

Give me a HUG:

I promise I don't bite!!:

Please dry my tears:

I weep not for me, but for you:

But most of all

Just love me for who I was, who I am, and who you think I have become, because

I AM STILL ME!!

THANK YOU ELAINE

The Angels knew what they were doing,

The day that you were born,

Every light went on in the world,

On that wonderful morn.

Through your life you have brought

Love and laughter, which so many sought;

Unending care, and always for others,

A wonderful wife and fantastic mother.

The world was blessed when you were born.

I will always be grateful, all my love, Norrm.

FIGHTING BACK!!

When your whole world collapses around you,

And everything you do is wrong,

When you're looking for someone to turn to,

And all you want to be is strong,

When dementia invades your life,

And seeps into every pore,

Its shakes both you and your wife

To the very core,

Please take a look around you,

At everything you've done,

You have so much more to do,

And so much more to come,

Pick up your sword and fight,

Family, friends and all,

Fight with all your might,

When Dementia comes to call!!

With help and huge support,

From everyone around

It will never breach your Fort,

You will never hear its sound.

I WONDER WHY?

 Wondering why it's always me,

Same old question, cannot see,

How much more do I endure?

Before they find that B****Y cure,

Every day, same old fight,

Pushing through with all my might,

But pushing through is what I do,

I`m sending all my love to you,

To all my family and all my friends,

One day I will be, on the mend

Will This Nightmare Ever End?

Crumbling walls within my brain,

Distant memories call my name,

Different days yet still the same

Will this Nightmare ever end?

 Not quite sure, what is real,

Forgetting how to eat a meal,

Desperation is what I feel,

Will this nightmare ever end?

All I want is to be alive,

I feel so old at Fifty Five,

My old age I want to see

Will this Nightmare ever end?

And so I walk with my illness

Hand in hand, my life amiss,

Waiting for cures elusive kiss

Will this nightmare never end?

Until that day, a cure is found,

You will always hear my sound,

Of defiance and hope abound,

Until my nightmare ends

Why Not Ask Me?

I`m still here, I can still speak,

I`m still strong, not frail and weak,

So when you stand there in my house,

Talking in whispers, just like a mouse,

Just look this way and you will see,

I`m still here, why not ask me?

Instead of saying, oh he can wear that,

And dressing me in some daft hat,

Or making me eat food I hate,

With me, why won't you debate?

I`m no different, can't you see,

I`m still here, I`m still me,

All I want is to have a choice,

All I want is to use my voice

Who Will Help Me Now?

You don't understand a word I say,

You don't understand my kind of day,

To be rid of this disease, is all that I pray,

Who Will Help Me Now?

All my family think I'm mad,

All my neighbours think I'm bad,

Yet deep inside I am so sad

Who Will Help Me Now?

Dementia takes away my hope,

It takes my knowledge of how to cope,

I feel I`m on a slippery slope,

Who Will Help Me Now?

Is this how I live for the rest of my life?

Seeing nothing but sorrow in the eyes of my wife,

Unknowingly causing this trouble and strife,

Who Will Help Me Now?

As every day passes I forget more,

Floating like flotsam, washed up on the shore,

Ever closer, to life's closing door,

Who Will Help Me Now?

I always wear, a happy mask,

Whilst struggling with every menial task,

So this time I`m going to ask,

Will YOU Help Me Now??

This last one was Written in the car on the way to Budleigh Salterton UK xxxxxxxx

BLOG   >>>>>>>>>>>>>>>>>>>>>>>>>

Lewy Body's and Hallucinations……. BE WARNED … VERY GRAPHIC

I have no memory of going to bed that night, and have very little memory of what happened after, apart from what I am about to tell you, but I have to warn you this is not for the faint heated or easily upset. What I am about to tell you, for the very first time, is the true Horrors of the hallucinations I have as best as I can remember. I will apologise now for the graphic nature of the writings but I feel I am at that stage of my disease I need to explain whilst I can, and as far as I know, il have never read anything like this, but, if you want to know the TRUE HORRORS of Lewy Body's dementia please read on, and if you have never heard of Lewy Body's dementia, please Google and have a look;

....

I stood frozen to the spot as I saw my attackers for the first time. They were all around me, their faces were made up of a million paper cuts, not bleeding heavily, but weeping droplets of blood. Their eyes were just slits with a blackness of the night emitting from them. They towered over me, about four of them, surrounding me and snarling from mouths that looked like chasms of sulphur with yellow protruding teeth, coming closer and closer every moment.

Suddenly one lashed out at me whilst screaming at I pitch I had never heard before, then they all attacked. Scratching me, ripping at my flesh, my arms burning at every cut, laughing and mocking me as they did so. I fought and I fought, I screamed like never before as I had trouble believing all that was going on around me. My flesh was hanging from my arms, my legs were torn to shreds, my stomach was hanging out as I tried, unsuccessfully, to push my insides back in again, until suddenly!! It stopped!! All I could hear was Elaine`s voice calming me, helping me move from the front room and back into my bed, stroking my face and whispering to me until eventually I fell asleep again.............. Or so I thought

The next thing I knew I was standing outside a lift (elevator). I could hear a child screaming and screaming, and as I looked across the room I was, in I saw a child's body, hanging out of a lift, trapped by the doors and the lift trying to drag her downwards into the abyss. I ran across, grabbed the child's hand and screamed for help, but nobody came, I wept. I sobbed as I saw her close her eyes as he slipped away from me down into the darkness. I had people all around me shooting abuse, some with knives as hands as they tried to take my life, trying all the time to hurt me as I screamed "What have I done wrong???

AGAIN, I AM BEING LED back to bed, this time from the kitchen by my ever loving Elaine, and so my night goes on, and hers I may add,

The time, 12.15am. We have only been in bed a couple of hours, and Elaine says sometimes this can go on all night!!! And it did do this night, but I can only remember what I have told you. The rest is lost to the dementia demon that is called Lewy Bod'ys type dementia.

FOOTNOTE

If ever anybody asks you what the difference is between Lewy Body's dementia and any other type, please tell them of this, and my quote is

'Having Lewy Body's Type dementia, rather than other types of dementia is like having

TWO TYPES OF DEMENTIA because, I have DEMENTIA, and KNOW I have dementia.'

I hope this helps and so sorry for the graphic nature of this.

END OF BLOG >>>>>>>>>>>>>>>>>>>>>>>>>>>>>>>>>>>>>

CHAPTER NINE

Doing Too Much

Well, the above sentence can be taken many ways my friends. Do I mean the person living with dementia doing too much, or the carer? Both are as important, but this time I mean the carer and when you think about it, I really would be the wrong person to lecture anybody about 'Doing Too Much' living with dementia LOL.

So what do I mean "Doing Too Much?" Whilst I really do believe that one of the rules right up there in the caring world is make sure you look after yourself, even if it is tinged with a bit of selfishness, because if you don't look after yourself, who`s going to look after us? After all, who CARES for the CARER? But what I would like to discuss here is actually doing TOO much for the person with dementia.

This may sound very strange to some as our natural instinct is to protect and care for our loved ones/patients, but sometimes you can actually CARE too much and inhibit what they do, thus they lose their lifestyle skills earlier and become less able much quicker than they normally would.

So, depending on what stage the person with dementia gets diagnosed, will depend on the abilities and tasks they can manage, but please don't be too quick to judge. In my own case of spatial awareness I cannot cross a road myself. My sense of danger has gone, and that little light/memory we spoke about on the Christmas tree has gone out. Yes I can sit here and tell you Man Vs. Bus, Bus will always win, and yet when I go to cross a road I will step straight out, so I need a full time carer with me at all times when I am out and about.

When in and around the house what can I and can't I do? I am not allowed to make a hot drink for many obvious reasons but that doesn't stop me helping with the washing up, sometimes the drying, folding clothes, helping making the bed, mixing by hand cake mixtures (not electrical) gardening, walking, dancing, singing and generally having a great time! As you can see there's a pattern forming here, my point is please don't start to do everything for those with dementia once they are diagnosed because they are more than capable of carrying on doing so much, once diagnosed, life doesn't end!! They are still the same person with the same past, same hobbies, likes and dislikes. The same things will still annoy them and the same things will also make them laugh. Yes, a diagnosis is devastating, but the last thing you need to feel on top of that is that you're on the scrap heap. In fact, if you are past retirement age I am a great advocator of doing more pastimes. Why not take up swimming, fishing, golf or any other leisurely pursuits you haven't done for years because you never had time?? It's not too late now to take up something new either!! I am a FIRM believer that the more you keep your mind occupied the more you can start to live with this awful disease and possibly even enrich your life, rather than just give up and let someone else do everything for you. As they say, the choice is yours, but the added benefit of this is if you can find things for the person with dementia to do so at clubs and social groups they will look after them for a couple of ours , then you will get that much needed break as well and a bit of DOWNTIME to do what YOU WANT!! It works both ways my friends!!

So now on to care homes, now this is a different kettle of fish but somewhere YOU could make a huge difference to people's lives. So many, many times are people admitted to care homes with the promise of full interaction on a regular basis, and so many times this does not happen. Please don't start shouting at me. If it does happen in your care home, if it does I will be the first to shout it from the rooftops and congratulate you all for all you do. But the fact is, it doesn't happen in as many as we would like. So let's get the political whinges out of the way first.

1. Not enough Staff

2. Wages are rubbish

3. Too much expected and not enough given back by management

4. Too many hours
5. Zero hours contract

And so on, all very valid and all good reasons for being upset about the way care homes are run, so if we know these things, and know the chances are, we have to live with things like this, then what are WE going to do about it??

We know there is no money about, Err, LIVE WITH IT

 We know, the country is run by (allegedly) Muppets, regardless of what party you belong to and we know, Err, LIVE WITH IT
We know the future isn't really as rosy as some would say it is, again Err, LIVE WITH IT

But what we DO KNOW is we can make a huge difference to people lives by just changing the smallest thing and it doesn't cost a penny.

To many times people are placed in care homes and they end up sitting in a (God forbid) wing backed chair, sat watching TV all day or listening to the radio and the only interaction is the odd walk by staff and mealtimes. For goodness sake, what do these people who run these places think these guys did before being placed in a care home? Do they think that all they ever did was sit around at home all day and fall asleep?? How ridiculous is that??

Most people who have been placed in care homes would have come from an environment of the kitchen, gardening, and everyday tasks we take for granted, so why should they stop? Why shouldn't all staff invite residents to help wash up, dry , lay the table cloth and table, pick flowers from the garden for the table, help make beds, cook, mix cake mixtures, bake cakes, under supervision? All these things are do-able as they say, just because they are in a care home doesn't mean they lose the use of their arms and legs, and it CERTAINLY doesn't mean they have stopped THINKING for themselves!! All these things can be implemented with little or no cost, all it takes is a little thought and understanding.

Another way to alleviate their boredom and make new friendships is to get to know your clients/resident's, (one day someone will come up with a name we all agree with lol).

Once you know their history, their likes/dislikes, previous occupations and hobbies you can arrange those with similar interests to sit next to each other. Introduce them, tell them how they both used to work in a factory, adored cooking, worked in a mill etc, or both love to do crosswords, scrabble and word search, you can see where I am going with this can't you? All it takes is a little effort and listening skills and you could enrich the lives of others immensely! All this can be done at NO COST whatsoever; all it takes is a little research by you.

Start a Bakery club and begin by asking all to write down their favourite recipe, once done you could gook a different recipe every week, who knows, you might even write a book on old recipes for all to follow at the home, the ideas are endless, but not hard or clever ideas, just common sense and a lot of understanding. All this can be done at a moment's notice as well, so simple, yet very effective. It's a team effort, and when you work it out, whilst the residents are busy playing cards, baking cakes, chatting about old times working in the mill and such, it will free you carers up to catch up on anything that needs doing?? Go on, give it a try.

BLOG >>>>>>>>>>>>>>>>>>>>>>

ONE DAY AT A TIME

Ten days ago I was at my absolute lowest. I/we had not slept for five days because of my hallucinations, and then continuous night terrors when I did get a couple of hours of sleep. A feeling of complete exhaustion because my CONCRETE OVERCOAT (my depression) lay so heavy across both body and mind. I cannot tell you how close I came to running away from it all, such is this awful terrible disease.

When we had a couple of days away all I kept saying to Elaine was "What are we going to do?" Elaine replied "About what darling?"

""EVERTHING" I kept shouting, "EVERYTHING !!" making no sense at all. When you have this disease, the red mist and black skies descend together sometimes making the 'perfect storm'. You feel like there is nowhere to turn, even trying talking to loved ones becomes so very difficult because you know how bad you feel, how low you are, but the words just won't come out!! Then there is the awful hidden fear of upsetting them. I was so very close to saying

"I CANT DO THIS ANYMORE"

It was only waking up two days ago, and only a day before a huge conference and Elaine's special night that I felt as if some of my concrete overcoat had been shed. On the day of the conference I was up early and knew that I had less than an hour to make my mind up as I really wasn't feeling that well. Even being driven to the conference I was still having "My Moments" and quite confused. The day did get better as time passed and by the time I stood and did my presentation I felt, once again like my old self and it went so very well.

The Awards night couldn't have gone any better and was, as you know, rounded off by my wonderful Elaine winning her award, but it could have been so very different, because this disease just doesn't care about conferences or awards ceremonies. It takes no prisoners, has no conscience or guilt and doesn't care whose lives it ruins. Truth be known, it feels like I/we got away with it this time, but what about the next and the next? Now you know why we advise people to take one day at a time with this illness, and cherish each day, each minute, each second, because things can change so very rapidly and without warning, and there is always a very real chance that one day I won't be able to claw myself back to reality, but until then, one day at a time, is ok by me

END OF BLOG >>>

Chapter 10

Picture's

To give you all a break from reading here's a few photos to look at, hope you enjoy

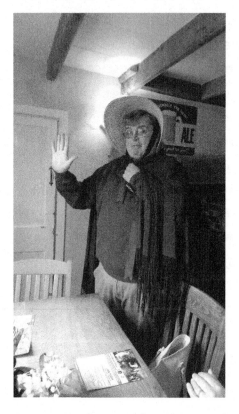

Oops, maybe not that one He he he

How about this one?

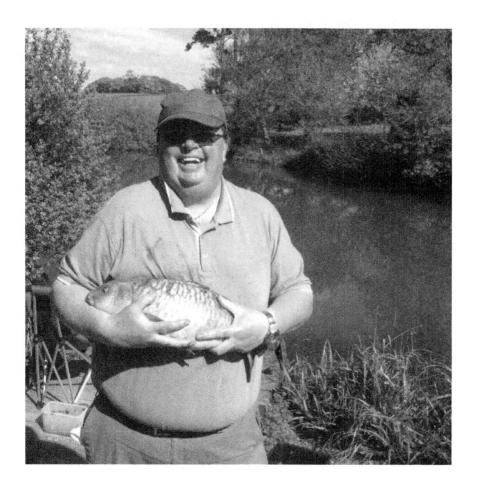

I have recently taken up coarse fishing at the grand old age of 58, and loving every minute of it. With the right carer there's not a lot you can't achieve when you put your mind to it.

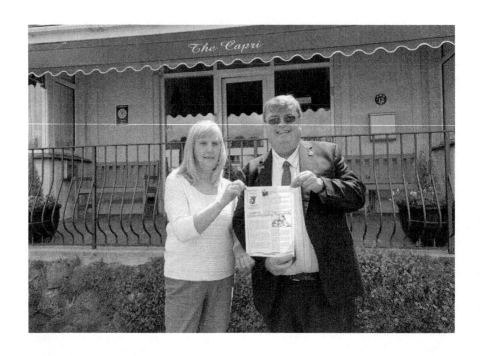

Awarding local Businesses' with purple Angel accreditation.

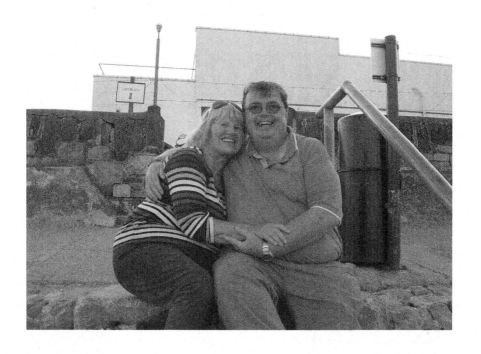

My Wonderful "Angel" Elaine and myself taking time out.

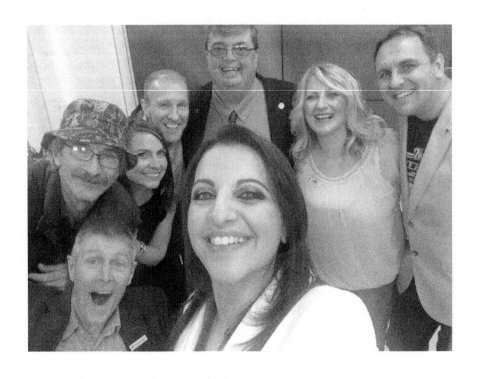

At Sky TV on the Chrissy B show.

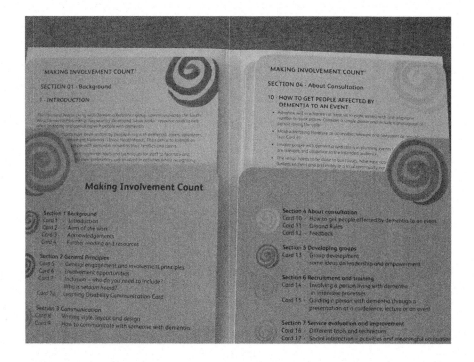

First piece of Major work I did with the Alzheimer's society UK and the incredible Anne Rollings.

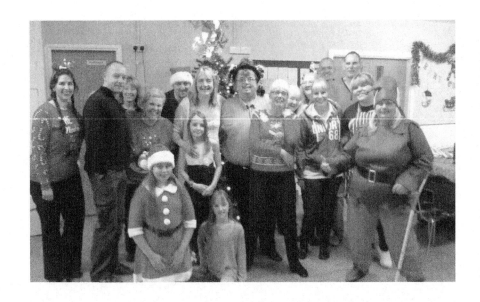

A Christmas dinner organised by Elaine and I for over 50
lonely people in Torbay, here are the Wonderful volunteers.

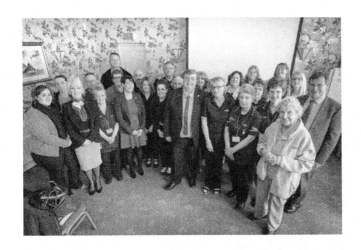

Doing what I love to do best, talking LOL

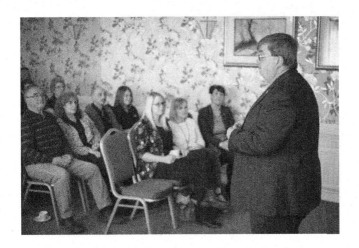

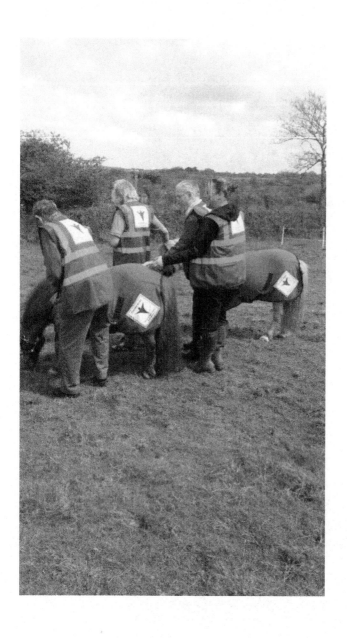

Purple Angel Ponies, thank you Angela Downing

xxxxxxxxxxxx

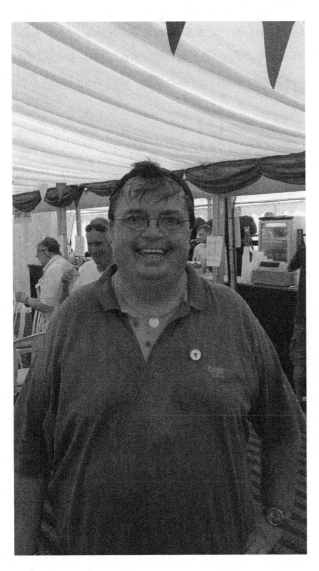

Proper geezer lol

Elaine and I at the Pride of Britain awards. I won the Pride of Britain Local hero award for the whole south west of the UK but didn't win the big one on the night, but hey ho, great night out in London.

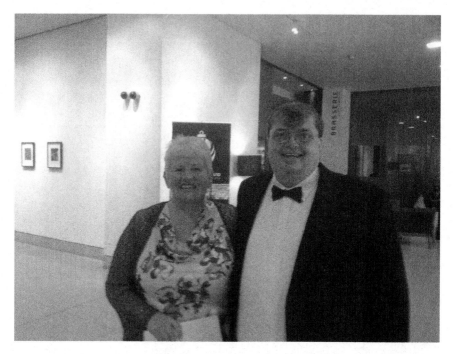

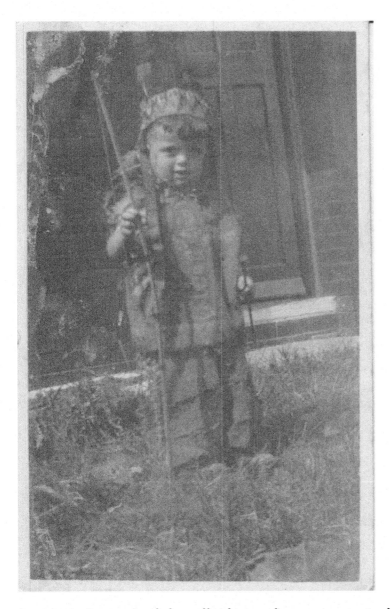

Last one, I promise lol, well, I have always supported the underdog!!

BLOG   >>>>>>>>>>>>>>>>>>>>>>>>>>>>>>>>>>>>>>>

Q. What does DEMENTIA feel like?

A. IT FEELS LIKE SOMETHING`S BROKEN

It feels like something's broken within my whole body, but I don't know what?

It feels like I have lost my very first teddy and cannot find it anywhere.

It feels like I had been picked to play football for the school team for the very first time, and just come down with flu.

It feels like I have just been dumped for the first time.

It feels like I have just lost my first wage packet on the way home from work.

It feels like waking up on a wet and windy morning knowing it could be the last thing you remember, never seeing, or remembering the sunshine again.

It feels like I was too late for the school trip and saw the bus full of my friends disappearing in the distance.

It feels like I have just been made redundant from my all-time favourite job.

It feels like I have just been stood up at the altar.

It feels like I have just lost someone, very close, for the very first time.

It feels like I am broken and cannot be fixed.

(Imagine feeling ALL of this at the same time, but a million times worse)

Q. What does dementia feel like??

A. ALL OF THE ABOVE and sadly much more

END OF BLOG   >>

Chapter 11

Choosing the right carer,

Now my friends, I have to say right at the start of this that regarding me having a carer just after I was diagnosed was a subject I wouldn't even discuss!! Me, aged 50 odd and having a 'Babysitter' as I called it then! NOT A CHANCE!!! You would not believe the arguments Elaine and I had over this. The rows, the silent moments and the tears, I am not ashamed to say. Elaine, my social worker, CPN (Community Psychiatric nurse) and my doctor all advised me to have one, but I stood firm for years and years, just flatly refusing one.

Then, one day, I looked into Elaine's eyes and she looked absolutely shattered. My heart sank as I realised there and then how selfish I had been. How could I do this to the only woman I have ever loved? I adore her and owe her so much! So it was time to swallow my pride and help her get some respite as well as begin, or at least try to, a new friendship with a carer. Elaine always promised that nobody would come through the door unless I invited them to; she said it was my choice and my choice only and would stand by my decision, so with that said we started the search. Please remember this was a few years ago and everybody is different depending at what stage they are at with their disease. Here goes……………………….

Carer number one

My everlasting impression of this chap was one of not only disbelief but also wondering to this day if he is still doing the same job!! Within 15 minutes, I kid you not, I was losing the will to live as he told me all about his wife who was manic depressive and I knew completely every tablet she took. He lasted 20 minutess before I asked him to leave!!

It didn't get much better for a while as carer after carer turned up and I sent them all packing within ten to fifteen minutes. Now, please don't get the idea that I am fussy or picky, let's see if you agree with me.

Is it really too much to ask that these people turn up for work clean shaven, tidy and presentable, and not looking like a cross between Grizzly Adams, Wurzul Gummage and smelling like a refuse yard ??? Elaine was just wonderful, and a lot politer than me as she showed them the door! I don't think I was as polite as I remember.

Then in came the Mexican!! He brought his lap top and sat in the front room for two hours whilst I sat in my bedroom on my computer! For me it was the perfect situation, I said hello and shut my bedroom door. Elaine went out for two hours, and then I said goodbye to him as he left two hours later, perfect! No not really as it only caused more arguments and the idea of having a carer went out of the window for a while. Then I decided to try again, I got someone from an agency here in Torquay who seemed quite chatty and quite alert and educated. The day came when it was decided I should bite the bullet and actually go out with them, in their car, in public! Now I know you are thinking this sounds very like a drama queen lol, but I was genuinely scared, and if you know me as my family do, that's something that very rarely happens.

I sat in the car in the car park wishing I was anywhere else. The destination, it was a meeting at the local Alzheimer's society office regarding a dementia leadership group. We set off, seat belt firmly on and went on our way; all was well until it came to parking the car. There was a space right outside where my appointment was and all he had to do was parallel park, yes? Err no!!! Five times he tried to park it!! He went up the kerb three times, was so close to getting hit by other oncoming cars until eventually coming to a stop on an angle. He let me get out of the car on my own, into oncoming traffic and it was only a miracle that stopped me from being hit. I asked him if he had just passed his test and he said he had been driving for years. All this was witnessed by Alzheimer's society staff, who were watching out of the window.

The time came for me to go home and he picked me up, not a word was spoken in the car but when we arrived back and Elaine asked what kind of day I had. I couldn't hold back any longer and it all came pouring out, but the best was yet to come! Elaine listened in horror of the events that had unfolded that day, she turned to him and said

"Is this TRUE?"

He looked her right in the eyes and said?

NO!!!!

He LIED, there and then, without a thought!! He said none of it was true and I was EXAGGERATING!! I was livid!! I screamed at him to get out of my house and have to say he was a very lucky man to only end up with a bruised ego. I cannot remember ever being so mad in my life!! It took Elaine ALL day, and more to calm me down. I was more annoyed he had lied to Elaine more than anything else and of course he was reported, and you wonder why I didn't want a carer? But things did get a lot better and I was introduced to John.

John was a happy chappy, a family man with a great sense of humour; he had to have as he was a Queens Park Rangers fan!! (sorry John, only joking) and he was only a few years younger than me. We hit it off straight away and we also both had a love of football and also sea fishing. So many trips were planned, had and enjoyed, and it wouldn't be the first time we have caught a full bag of mackerel, sat on the bus on the way home and asked "Can you smell fish ???" he he.

Alas after about a year John decided he wanted to better himself and went for a promotion, and quite rightly so. He was a family man, and as someone who has always said family and health must come first he had my full backing along with a letter of recommendation, but, as you can guess I was back to square one. As it was winter we decided to leave it until the better weather and try again, this is what happened next…………………..

Once again we decided to go with agency workers and the first one walked in, unkempt, unshaven and well, I can't say much more for fear of being sued. The second, well, he walked in very well spoken, very smart and quite educated so it looked promising, all I asked was if they knew how to fish, especially coarse fishing, as I wanted someone to teach me. I was assured this was the case and a date was made to go to Exeter canal for a day of lure fishing.

The morning came and he turned up. He was wearing a Crombie coat (big expensive woollen knee length coat) suit pants, desert shoes, beige, and a shirt and tie!! Now I know I said smart and casual, but HEY GUYS we were going fishing for goodness sake!!! I said nothing, Elaine tried not to laugh and off we went. The journey was about twenty minutes and was quite jovial. We arrived, unloaded the car and set the chairs and fishing rods up. It was only after a couple of minutes I heard the noises coming from him, teeth chattering and a flapping of arms, beating himself trying to keep warm, this didn't bode well at all, but it was all I could do not to laugh in his face. It wasn't cold and was about 16c. I got my line tangled and asked him for help. He looked at me as if I had just asked him to explain the theory of relativity and obviously knew nothing about fishing!! Thankfully a fisherman was passing by and he helped me.

Within ten minutes he announced that he was going for a walk up the canal to get warm?? So I announced to him, what part of "you are my carer and have to make sure I am safe at all times, especially so close to water", didn't he understand? Outcome, another silent ride home and another goodbye.

Please meet Peter, my carer now.

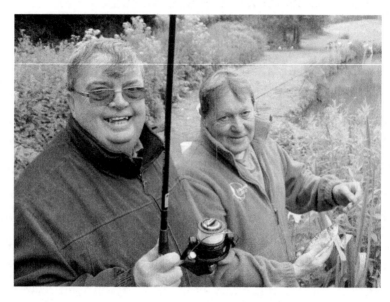

As you can see we are stood side by side having a great time fishing, and we have actually caught a few !!

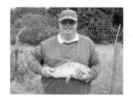 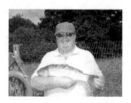 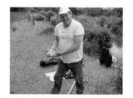

Peter is without doubt the best carer to date, why? Because the wonderful guys at Bluebird Care in Torbay listened to what we wanted and matched us up. He is around my age, spent years fishing, is a football fan, has a great sense of humour and is a laid back fellow. Plus has all he needs to be a carer, a good listener and empathetic to others less fortunate than him, and this is my point.

When you are looking for a carer, you certainly don't have to take the first one that comes along, or because you will feel awful telling them they don't suit. Think about the persons likes, dislikes, hobby's, food favourite's. Do they like to go out, and to where? Or would they rather stay in playing cards or dominoes etc. Age range can also be so important, please make sure they are comfortable with the age and the sex of the carer. Write all these down and approach different care companies to get the best, and most suitable not only to them, but to you as well. Remember to talk about hours etc.

Most of all, please remember, you and the person with dementia are in charge. You are effectively employing someone to work with you. The one thing I MUST INSIST on is you must INSIST yourself that you get the SAME carer every time except for illness and holidays, which cannot be helped. If they can't accommodate this, then move along to the next care company, and the next, and the next, until they do.

Once you have done this and both built not just a rapport but also a friendship, the benefits will become all too clear.

A good carer is someone who will walk side by side with you and the person with dementia. They will open car doors for you and make sure there is no traffic coming. It's a person who will go the extra mile and will take no notice of others when they stare and point and they will, believe me. A good carer is someone who will ring up before they arrive and remind you to make sure they have a hat and sun tan lotion when it's a warm sunny day, but most of all a carer is someone like my carer called Peter who once said to me,

" The Clue is in the name CARER"

This chapter would not be complete without mentioning my MATE Trevor who is my good friend, Karen's husband. When I didn't have a carer, when nobody else seemed to care or wanted to go fishing with me, Trevor did!! We spent many an hour on Exeter canal lure fishing and he is the only man I know who can fish two rivers at once!! (private joke). Did we catch anything?? Did we heck, but we caught plenty of mackerel when we went sea fishing so that more than made up for it. Karen and Trevor, you will always be in our hearts xxxxxxxxxxxx

ANOTHER TIME, ANOTHER DAY

As we travelled back to Torquay from Newton Abbot, I got a message on my phone. I looked down, read it, and answered straight back, but as I looked up I wasn't where I thought I was. On the left of me we were just passing the Salvation Army hostel, the Clarence Pub was up on the right and at the bottom of the road was the junction where Gordon's garage sat, I was on TOPP WAY in Bolton Lancs.

"Why are we in Bolton, and how did we get here?" I asked Elaine who does all the driving. She glanced across at me with that very worried look on her face, "we are not in Bolton love" she said, "We are on our way back to Torquay!!"

"Yea right I laughed, well how come we are on TOPP Way, Bolton then?" "We are not darling, we are in Devon". The look on her face said it all, the sadness, the sorrow, and the slight look of fright as she knew I was having 'One of my moments'. I shook my head and looked back down at my phone. Maybe I am dreaming I thought and closed my eyes, expecting to wake in bed beside the love of my life and it had all been a dream, but I didn't, because as I looked up again, Gordon's garage was coming ever closer on the Junction of Topp Way and Higher Bridge street Bolton. I clenched my fist in frustration as something at the back of my mind was telling me there was something very wrong, but I could see what I could see and nobody else could tell me any different!!!!

 Then, as quick as it all happened, the scenery around me changed, and I was suddenly back in REAL TIME, sat in the passenger seat, just passing Tesco's on the left hand side in Newton Abbot Devon, and all was back to normal (if you can call it that). We pulled into the car park and sat there in complete silence, trying to make sense of what just happened. It was just two thirty in the afternoon, not a good sign. Eventually Elaine took my hand and whispered, Don't worry, all will be ok, and all was well with the world again, well, for the time being.

This is one awful cruel disease, and I know deep down, there will come a time when I will not be able to differentiate between the realty of everyday life and hallucination's, but until that day arrives, I promise I will do my best to share these happenings with you for as long as I can, much love my friends,

END OF BLOG   >>>>>>>>>>>>>>>>>>>>>>>>>>>>>

CHAPTER 12
Purple Angel Music

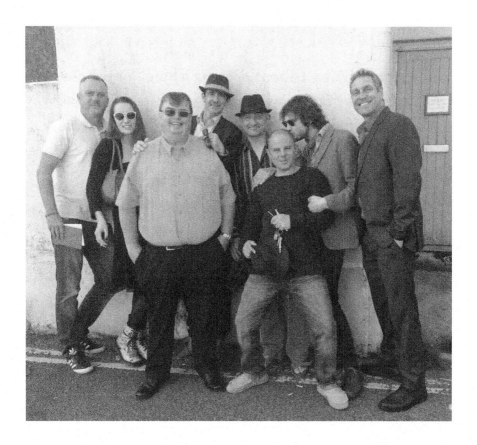

I have to say this has to be one of my all-time favourite pictures outside of Ocean Studios, Paignton with Ashley Sims, Barney Dine, Michael Campari, Hannah Leach, Micky Pig and Alex Mc Ginnes. This is what Purple Angel Music is all about, I will explain…………………………………..

Thanks to a dear friend Karen Jones and hubby Trevor, they introduced us to a certain Ashley Sims of Torquay, originally of Derby. Have you ever met someone for the first time and thought we are really going to get on?? This was one of those times and it doesn't happen that often in a lifetime.

We originally chatted about opening a hotel for people to come and have holidays with respite for carers but that quickly blossomed into Purple Angel Holidays which are NOW based in already existing prestigious hotel`s in Torbay, and from there we went from strength to strength.

The five day or so holidays we offer gives the carer so much needed respite as we will provide the activities, with a coordinator, for a few hours, three days a week in the afternoon so they can go off and have some 'Me Time' be it swimming, sunbathing, shopping or whatever. It's not care but it will give them that much needed break if they want to, here's a few details

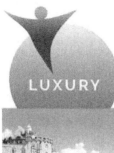

Purple Angel Holidays

Thank you for your booking

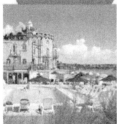
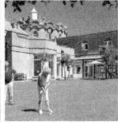
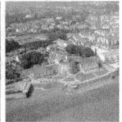

We are pleased to confirm your 'Luxury' holiday.

Thank you for booking with Purple Angel Holidays.
We are pleased to confirm your Luxury holiday.
We strive to provide great holidays for people living
with dementia and their carers. Let our Angels look
after your loved one for four hours per day, while you
relax and enjoy our beautiful Devon scenery. More
importantly, you will have the opportunity to meet other
carers and share your experiences.
You will be staying at the Redcliffe Hotel. Situated
close to the both Paignton and Preston Beaches, the
Redcliffe Hotel enjoys panoramic views over Torbay
and has three acres of grounds.

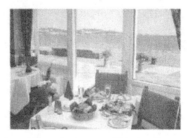

Directions to The Redcliffe Hotel

Directions
From Newton Abbot
At the Penn Inn roundabout take the 2nd exit (A380 signposted to
Torquay)
At the Kerswell roundabout take the 2nd exit (A380 Hamelyn Way)
At the next roundabout, take the second exit (Kings Ash Way)
At the next roundabout, take the first exit (Preston Down Road)
Carry on all the way down this road to the traffic lights
Keep in the left hand lane, going straight on to the seafront
Bear right with the road and continue along the seafront
The Redcliffe Hotel is on the left hand side, just after the two zebra
crossings

Paignton railway station, with main line services, less than a mile away
From Totnes
Head in to Paignton town centre then follow signs to the seafront
At the Apollo cinema turn left and continue along the seafront
The road bends sharply right then left past the Redcliffe Lodge Hotel
The Redcliffe is on the right hand side just past the Travelodge

There is a wealth of information on our website. If you need to
contact us, please phone on 01803 21 22 23 and our staff will be
pleased to help you.
Karen and the other Purple Angels look forward to seeing you.

The Redcliffe Hotel, Marine Drive, Paignton, Devon TQ3 2NL.

Telephone Number: 01803 21 22 23   Website: www.purpleangelsholidays.co.uk

When I first met Ash he was very honest and very upfront. He explained he knew nothing about dementia and asked me to explain it to him in layman's terms, which I did, re the Christmas tree lights analogy. I also explained that in the USA some research had been done which suggested that the receptor in the brain that received the signals of music when played was never affected by dementia, and that's why, even if you have dementia or not, you can always remember where you were, or who you were with when you hear a certain song from your past. A moment passed, and then Ash looked at me and said

"Why Don't You Sing To them? "

I have often said this is where our friendship and his brilliant ideas started to come together. "What do you mean?" I asked, he just said "I have an idea, leave it with me and I will get back to you". True to his word, two weeks later we met up and he showed me a prototype of his idea which was an MP3 that actually reminded people when to eat, drink, lock the door, turn the fire off etc. My first words were it's the craziest, maddest thing I have ever heard of, but within seconds, the realization of how many people this could help began to dawn on me and another dementia aid was born, and happy to say, looks like being very successful. Please see information

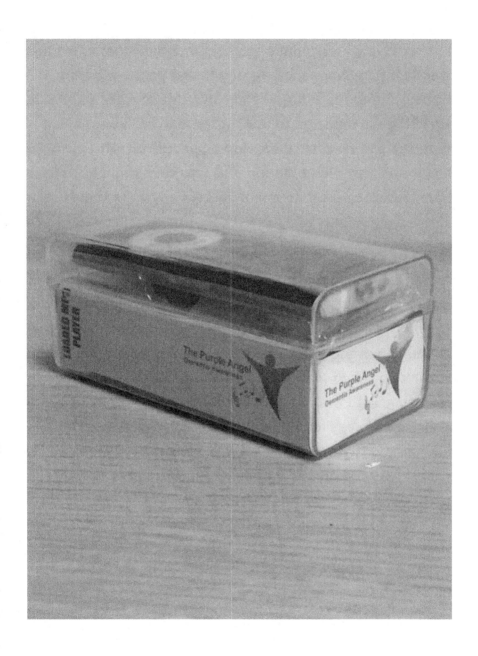

More Info of the Purple Angel Music can be found on its
website which is   http://www.purpleangelmusic.co.uk/

So there we were, happily hatching out new ideas when the weirdest thing happened. Ashley took a phone call from trading standards in Buckinghamshire, of all place`s and said we had been reported to trading standards. Someone had reported us saying we were ripping people off with the MP3 players as they didn't work?? This was very strange at the time, because, we hadn't actually sold any up to then!!

Then things got even stranger!! They, (Trading standards) asked us what we did and when we said (well, actually Ashley said) he invents things to help people. Trading standards said it would be brilliant if we could invent something that would stop people being scammed over the phone and at their own doorstep, so guess what? We did!!! So, actually from that 'TROLL' (politest word I can think of) reporting us to trading standards on some trumped up claim, we were given the idea of the doorbell tunes and phone apps that remind you not to give out your bank details over the phone and stops scammers in their tracks when they come to your door asking to 'tarmac your drive Sir' and so forth. Funny how life works out isn't it?? As Elaine always says, out of something bad comes something good and it did!!

Details

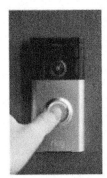

PURPLE ANGEL
DEMENTIA AWARENESS

Purple Angel Music Door Bell

Purple Angel Music have been working closely with trading standards after they asked us to help fight door step and phone scammers, targeting the elderly and the vulnerable. We have created two products designed specifically to help deter these people, it is not a cure but we feel this is the best thing on the market right now.

Door Bell: we can supply and install a fully working door bell with one of our specially written MP3s that suggests that the house is in no need of any home repairs or improvements, this is something that hopefully would create concern from the canvasser that the house has additional protection and cause them to move on.

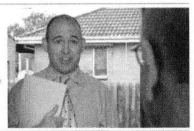

Purple Angel Music Ring Tones

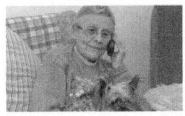

Phone ringtone: most phone scammers ask for donations for bogus charities or inform the person that they have won the lottery and just require a payment from them to release the money, the song, which is an old nursery rhyme or hymn emphasises mainly "don't give out your bank details" and also " don't give out your card details, it is also possible to have a motion sensor installed next to the phone which maintains the tune playing even after the phone has been picked up, all gentle intro music and familiar tunes designed specifically not to scare the person living on there own but hopefully put off the caller and make them move on. This product is available now for mobile phones, the motion sensor is ready now and we will be sourcing a MP3 uploadable land hand set mid 2016.

Website: www.purpleangelmusic.co.uk

I have to say working with, and still working with Ashley Sims, Keith Byron and co is an absolute pleasure and I am sure will continue to be in the upcoming future. One thing I am certain of is there is much more to come, and I just can't wait.

BLOG   >>

NEITHER HERE NOR THERE ………………….PLEASE SHARE

Sitting there in early evening I was transported to another place, my eyes are wide open, so I am not dreaming. In this 'other place' I have appointments, things to do, and know many people, but when I am back 'here' as I call it, I cannot name anybody or anywhere I have just been.

Whilst I am 'THERE' I seem to be living an alternate life. The people I meet, talk to and even work with I feel I have known for years, and when I am 'Back' here, I know nothing of who they are. I feel an emptiness within as if I am missing out on things. I have that edgy feeling as if I should be somewhere, or I have missed an important meeting and shouldn't be 'HERE' sometimes. I really hope this is making some kind of sense to you all, as even I am having trouble explaining this!

My memory is not good anyway as you can imagine, I mean, don't get me wrong, it could be a lot worse as I have Lewy Body disease and not Alzheimer's as first thought, but where as in 'REAL LIFE' as I call it, I forget completely many things, and yet, the scant memories of being 'OVER THERE' are like being in a sky of clouds and every now and again the clouds break and I just catch a glimpse of what may, or may not have just happened. I am told this happens when I am hallucinating, and yet, my hallucinations are usually of terrible things happening to family and friends, awful deadly things which I wouldn't even discuss with my Angel Elaine, but this, this is like everyday life, and very real to me, and yet it's not!!

Is this me slipping ever forward into the ABYSS?? Is this what happens when people with dementia tell you stories of where they have been, what they have been doing and who with, even though you know it's not really happened. I believe these are not hallucinations as such, or as I know them anyway, but the mind playing tricks on me, and others, because of my/their dementia symptoms. I believe the two are totally separate!! Either way, none are very nice and certainly NONE ARE WANTED!!

What do you think??

END OF BLOG

>>>

Chapter 13

WRAD

World Rocks Against dementia 2016

Well, this was billed as my swansong to all as it's without a doubt the BIGGEST thing Elaine and I had ever attempted. I have to say RIGHT FROM THE START if it wasn't for friends, family, steering groups, and a WRAD Committee we would never have managed it, but this is how it all started.

In 2015 I came across someone called Wayne Mesker from the USA on Facebook who had started something called 'Rock Against dementia' which I thought was such a good idea. Now I, being a HUGE music lover just loved this idea and suggested we did something both here and in the states. I asked if I could use his fantastic logo and incredibly he said not only YES but invited me to coordinate the Purple Angel logo in it. Rock against dementia 2015 was a forerunner of things to come in 2016. It was held in a local pub here in Torquay, in some places in Wales by my dear welsh friends, and a few places around the world, but only very small events, little did we know what was to come in 2016

WRAD 2016 started to live and breathe all on its own. Every day we got emails from all over the world asking how could they join in and we soon found that if we didn't get organised, and fast, it would overwhelm us very quickly.

Before we knew it we had offers from the wonderful incredible Music Mill in Newton Abbot run by Ali and Lenny (I had worked with them previously on a song I wrote for an event in Torquay).Then came along Samantha Montini, an incredible singer, her mum, a fantastic volunteer, bookkeeper and secretary, Lisa Doran, a friend of many years and HEY PRESTO!! We had a team!! I remember the first meeting we ever had, we just sat there, looking at each other thinking errrr, what's next?? LOL. I explained to all the interest we had had from a couple of countries and how I had a feeling it was maybe going to get a little bigger. Little did I know that sentence would come back and bite me on the bum, in a nice way?

We looked at some venues and thought about it a bit more. Eventually the venue we decided on was the English Rivera Centre, on Chestnut Way Torquay. The first time we met there was hardly a sound that came from our mouths, it was ABSOLUTLY HUGE!! I just stood there trying to take it all in, I have to admit at this point I just wanted to turn and run. It was a 1,000 + seater, with the biggest and deepest stage I had ever seen and the full enormity of what we were attempting swept over all of us. We sat and ordered coffees for all, and silence once again was the winner for a short time.

Eventually, one of us said, I can't remember who,

So, here we are then!!

We all collapsed with laughter, took a deep breath and decided to get on with the job in hand. I won't bore you with all the details but a few months later and after a lot of hard work, tears, a few tantrums and a lot of sleepless nights (and that was just me LOL) we ended up with this

25+ countries involved
Events all over the world happening on the same day at the same time, (Time zones allowing) Thousands of people across the globe coming together as one with a simple message
'Together we are strong'

We even had China dancing in the aisles and all wearing Purple Angels (even Bob Geldof didn't get China during his famous LIVE AID spectacular!) and I will use that TAGLINE for years to come!! We, in Torquay, had a 12 hour music and entertainment extravaganza which included so many different choirs, artists, both young and old and then two super groups (in my eyes), in the evening being the incredible LIONSTAR and the SIMMETONES.

At 2.30pm exactly in the afternoon the incredible Plymouth Military wives came on stage, all dressed in Purple and looking beautiful, each and every one of them. Their musical producer Rob Young also looking great (he will never forgive me if I don't say that LOL) and singer, tenor Tyrone Phillip Roth Piper also took to the stage. That day HISTORY WAS MADE. They began to sing a song called 'Within My Mind' which I wrote myself and the wonderfully clever Rob Young had written the music to.

The song itself started out as a poem which I had written for my darling wife Elaine, the original Purple Angel. I showed it to a great friend of mine and who is also a Plymouth Military wife singer Kristy Ann Johnson who suggested it would make a great song and knew just the person who might write the music for it, that person being Rob Young no less. Within a couple of months we were round at Robs, jamming (as you do lol) and a song was born. On top of that the wonderful, brilliant, Larraine Smith and the Plymouth Military wives said they would sing it on the day, so the scene was set.

Have you ever had a dream that you have organised a party and no one turns up?? Well, you can imagine what we all felt on the morning of WRAD, a new ERA, a HUGE 1,000 seater to be filled and having never done anything like this before. Two things kept popping into my head;

1. The Blues Brother's film where they had no idea how many would turn up till the day?

2. The Kevin Costner film Fields of Dreams, famous for 'If you build it they will come'

I am so happy to say both applied. By the time 2pm came that day you couldn't get a seat and we had to open upstairs for more seating. As the Plymouth military wives' walked on and Tyrone started singing you could hear a pin drop. It was just one of the magical moments I will, hopefully, never forget, along with the rest of the day and I am so happy to say that because it was so successful ADI, (Alzheimer's Disease International), have now taken it on and the event will be held every year around the world. They do say fortune favours the brave, and I have to agree, especially because Kirsty Johnstone is organising the next one in Devon, good luck dear friend, here's some pictures.

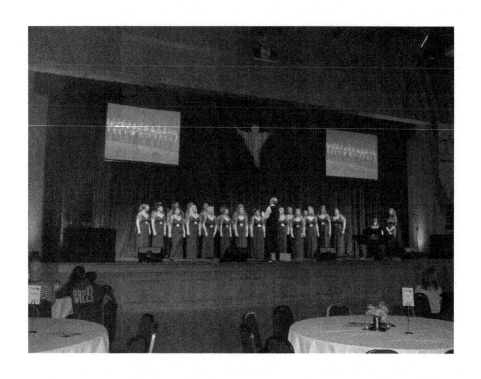

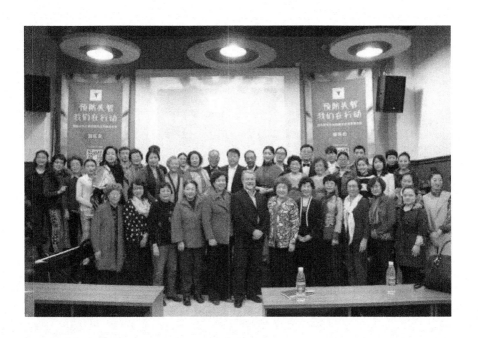

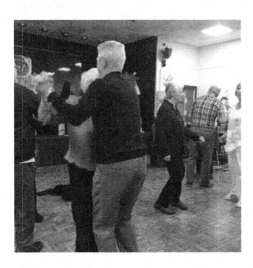

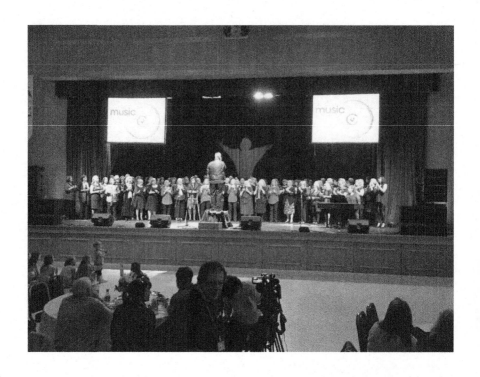

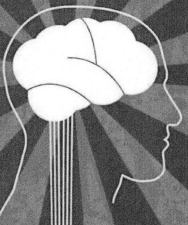

ROCK
AGAINST

DEMENTIA

PURPLE
ANGELS

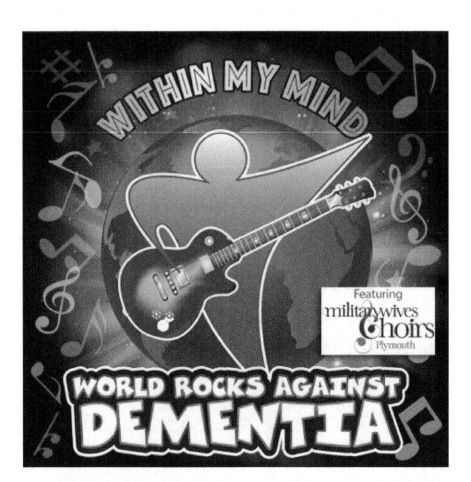

BLOG   >>>>>>>>>>>>>>>>>>>>>>>>>>>>>>>>>>

Changing the Face of Conferences'

I have, over the years, spoken at many conferences, though I may not be invited to do so again after writing this, but I am, after all 'Supposedly retired', but hey ho!! But there has always been one question on my lips and more so lately, and that is, after all the back slapping, statistic`s unveiled and being sold different assistive appliances,

WHAT HAPPENS NEXT???

Now I am not talking about the DAI (Dementia Alliance International) or Alzheimer's Disease International who recommend polices to the World Health Organisation (WHO), but other`s around the UK and the World. For years we have campaigned to have more people LIVING WITH Dementia invited to these conferences, and in recent times this has happened I am glad to say, but I am talking about what happens AFTER the conference is over, the floors swept, and tables cleared and put away?

Yes we have people writing on white boards, idea trees, post it notes and discussions around tables, BUT WHAT

THEN? How this is translated to the shop floor so to speak and is it EVER turned into an action?

When was the last time you went to a conference and 12 months later you stood there and said to yourself WOW we discussed this at the conference last year and now it's happening, my quality of life is so much better now!

Answers on a postcard please!!

The point I am trying to make is what's the point of these things if it isn't turned into actual living, walking, life enhancing actions?? It's ok to collate all the ideas and number crunch, but if it doesn't benefit others, what's the point?? In this day and age of social media and video conferences any type of information is available at the touch of a keyboard, so why do we need to spend (dare I say) monies that could be better spent on real life services, memory cafes and other much needed things? As they say in the song, it's NOT really about the money, it's about the fact that hundreds of people turn up, have their say, meet old friends, compare notes and then go home after having a 'Jolly Good Time' and then forget about it until the next one!!!

Now, if I had my way, and in my humble opinion it would happen like this……………………………..

Action plans would be made up from differing parts of the conferences, not just the best ones picked but also the very practical and simple to apply ones. Then a reasonable timeline given (these things don't happen overnight) and then the team in charge of implementing it must be held accountable if not acted upon, it's not really rocket science is it??

Am I by myself in thinking this? I would love to know?

What we need is action, for too long now we have had 'Blah Blah Blah' and a lot of hot air and promises. Let's set "To Do By" dates, let's turn plans into actions and let's improve lives for ALL those touched by Dementia. Please share (especially with heads of Dementia organisations and conference organisers), and please let me know what you think.

The next time YOU attend a conference, please always ask the organizer at the end

Q. So, now what are YOU going to do about it ??????

END OF BLOG   >>>>>>>>>>>>>>>>>>>>>>>>>>>>>>>>>>>>>

Chapter 14

Nearly There,

As I write these last few pages I can feel the emotions welling up inside of me. It's a very strange thing to write and say goodbye, even though most of the time I feel reasonably ok, but truth is the truth and dementia is a terminal disease. No lies, this book has been hard to write but I hope in years to come it will be used to show the world that there is LIFE AFTER DIAGNOSIS and being diagnosed doesn't mean the end of everything. I cannot state how important an early diagnosis is and how, if given, can open up, rather than close some roads.

As I come to the closing pages of this book I have to say that in the past there have been doubters, shall we say, and there have been lots of hills to climb and lots of questions to answer. I will be the first to say, I didn't get it right all the time, nobody ever does, and if they think they do, they are fools, but I would like to think I tried my best.

There is one thing I will never do and that's to apologise for doing so well for so long!!! That's like asking someone with cancer why they have lived for 20 years when they were only given 5!!

Yes, I have lost count of how many times I have been asked

"How come you look no different than two years ago?" or "How come a member of my family died after only three years from being diagnosed?" For both of these questions I have no answer, just like I have no answer from myself as to why I have managed so well so far. But, there's one thing for sure, I will never say sorry for living with my dementia thus far. My time will come, no doubt, and when it does, I hope the last thing on my mind is the names of all my family and friends, (REAL FRIENDS) who have helped me on my way and helped us achieve what we have achieve, and long may it continue.

Can I just say to all carers/caregivers out there

"The Care You Walk Past, Is the care you accept,

STOP WALKING PAST!! "

To all Dr`s and Consultants

Get your act together, do not be afraid to diagnose and please remember, there is not a consultant or professor in the world that can tell me what those in late stages are thinking, even if they have lost mobility and speech. Just because they stop speaking doesn't mean they go deaf at the same time!!

Please don't be afraid of diagnosing a patient with dementia. If one of your patients walks into your surgery and complains of chest pains, you think heart problems, if they complain of nose bleeds and horrendous headaches you think aneurisms, if they have had a rapid weight loss for no reason you think cancer, and YET... ! Sometimes when people come into your surgery that you have known for a while and are quite clearly confused and unwell, you don't diagnose dementia??WHY PLEASE ??

To all family members and friends of those who know someone with dementia.

Just because they do not remember you anymore, doesn't mean to say, YOU don't remember them! It's them with the dementia, NOT YOU.

To all those who work in Public places.

When you see someone acting out of the ordinary, or doing something that seems so unlikely, just imagine yourself doing the very same thing, but you have no control over what you are doing and have no say in your actions. How would you feel deep down? It's really not their fault but the fault of their dementia.

As you know I am not particularly political (mind you the BREXIT was quite good fun discussing that LOL) But it's a well-known fact that the dementia charities/research etc, only get ONE EIGHTH of the funding that Heart, Cancer and Brain Tumour charities research get, but please remember this………………

I have met someone who has had major heart problems and survived.

I have met someone who had Cancer and survived.

I have met someone who has had a brain tumour and survived.

I have NEVER YET MET someone who has had Dementia and SURVIVED!!!!!!

Food for thought I think??

So, the time has come to say goodbye to one and all. Over the next few pages will be an up to date list of all Purple Angel Ambassadors and the countries we are established in, (Up to and including the date 21/07/2016). If you joined us after, or for some reason cannot see your name on here, please take it up with Jane Moore... LOL LOL!

My dear friends, on the back of this book I quote that it will be last sentence that will be the hardest one to write, but thankfully that's not because of my dementia, but it feels like I am saying a final goodbye.

It has been an absolute HONOUR and pleasure to know you all, work with you all, laugh with you all and cry with you all, and as always
Stay healthy, Stay happy , but most of all
STAY FRIENDS

See you all on the other side

Norrms

Norrms Mc Namara

List of Current Ambassadors

Norman McNamara, Torbay, Devon UK

Jane Moore, Camelford, Cornwall, UK

Anita Moran, Wrexham, N.Wales, UK

Chris Hodge, Johnstown, Wrexham, Wales, UK

Chantelle Merritt, Abingdon, Oxford, UK

Gary Joseph LeBlanc, Florida USA Head of Ops

Harry Urban, Pennsylvania, USA Head of Ops

Shari Felker, Santa Rosa Beach, Florida USA

April Lewis, Weston Super Mare, UK

Martina Kaut, Furtwangen, Germany. Head of Ops

Kim Monery, Chichester, W.Sussex, UK

Sandy Spencer Whelan, New Albany, Indiana, USA

Linda Finnigan, Motherwell, Scotland

Kathy Broggy, Knoxville, Tennessee, USA

Bridie Breen, Prestwich, Manchester, UK

Carol Bevin, Warrington, Cheshire, UK

Jennifer Mullin, Warrington, Manchester, UK

Dawn Smith, Newton-le-Willows, Merseyside, UK

John Kelly, Merseyside, UK

Barbara Clarke, Bolton, UK.

Sandy Williams Spencer, Arizona, USA

Joan Best, Halewood, Liverpool, UK

Mary Howard, Lititz, Pennsylvania, USA

Sue Stimpson, Kingston Upon Hull, Yorks. UK

Tony Hall, Bristol, UK

Linda Morse, Beerwah, Queensland,Australia

Ajay Chhetri, Kathmandu, Alzheimer's Nepal H of Ops

Rupak Rijal, Jhapa, Nepal H of Ops

Azizul Haque, Dhaka, Alzheimer's Bangladesh

Tracy Edwards Was Muirhead, Plymouth, Devon, UK

Jean Saunders, Shepperton, Middlesex, UK

Rowena Wilson, Bude, Cornwall, UK

Ann Collins, Bolton, UK

Kirsty Elgar, Minehead, Somerset, UK

Mick Sykes, Queensland, Australia

Stanton O Berg, Fridley, Minnesota, USA

June K Berg, Fridley, Minnesota, USA

Caron Sprake, Exeter, UK

Michael Ellenbogen, Pennsylvania, USA H of Ops

Mandy Rowlands, Hampshire, UK

Kenneth Jones, Liverpool, UK

*Susan Cornish, USA

Lori la Bey, Minnesota USA Head of Ops

Alison Smith, Illinois, USA

Bill Wilson, N Wales, UK

Hilary Cragg Torquay, UK

Zoe Fairburn, Plympton, UK

Sean Gale, Plymouth, UK

Sue Barlow, Reading, UK

Kim Pennock, Ebberston, UK

Kirstyanne Heath, Torquay, UK

*Samantha Beesley, Australia

Jackie Stuckey, Chesham, UK

Olivia Jones, Dorchester, UK

Stacie Jane Culloty, Little Chalfont, UK

Julie Meldrum (Element), Herefordshire, UK

Wanda Montgomery, Georgia, USA

Dishard bin Hussein, Colombo, Sri Lanka

John David Baker, Cheshire, UK

Karen Baker, Cheshire, UK

Philip Choban, Cluj Napoca, Romania

Carmen Almasan, Cluj Napoca, Romania

Jessica Reid, Exeter, Devon, UK

Pamela Goodwin, Mount Nasura, W.Australia

Sharon Connolly, Tauranga, New Zealand Head of Ops

Louise Ann Howard Batemans Bay, NSW

Tabitha Kay, Ontario, Canada

Cher Riley-Hart, Melksham, Wiltshire, UK

Lisa Holland, Olinda Trust, N.Wales, UK

Lisa Greaves, Middx, UK

Vitaliy Kravchenko, Ukraine

Ann Farr, Shotton, Flintshire, UK

Angee Turnbull, Canada

Julie Yates, St. Helens, Merseyside, UK

Pearl Weepers, Glenrothes, Scotland (UAE)

George Weepers, Glenrothes, Scotland

Max Wallack, Massachusetts, US

Jami Denmark, Washington, USA

Carrie Chan, Redhill, Singapore KYDZ Int. HofOps

Andrew Clark Hall, Nevada, USA

Laurie Mantz, Rhode Island, USA.

Jan Brummell, Queensland, Australia

Phil Redington, Bristol, UK

Hanna Idous, Morocco

Ann-Marie Harmer, Cambridgeshire, UK

Reena Ghale, Rochester, Kent, UK

Lisa Davis, Worcestershire, UK

Dr Ina Gilmore, Marion, Sth Carolina, USA

Sue Stratton &Harwich Nurses, Essex, UK

Sailesh Mishra, Silver Innings, India

Andrew Hall, N. Devon, UK (Now USA)

Illeana Santana, Connecticut, USA

Kammy Bennett, Bude, UK

Helga Rohra, Munchen, Germany

Beverley Hickey, Essex, UK

Janet Pitts, Oklahoma, USA

*Emma Aspden,

Lisa Houlihan, Devon, UK

The Fox Valley Memory Project, Wisconsin, USA via

Professor Susan Mcfadden and John

Kate Maggs, Gtr Manchester, UK

Alina Williams MSc, Trinidad & Tobago

Sandra & Harry Clarke, Dubai, UAE

Tamas Tatai, Hungary Head of Ops

Michael Jacobsen, Thailand.

Vivienne Davies-Quarrell, ace-alzheimers.comDenbighshire, UK

*M. Bally Singh, Royal Gdns., California

Gemma Blackmore-Cattran, Plymouth, UK

 Colleen Evans, Plymouth, UK

Shannen Garner, Suffolk, UK

Natasha Endean, Cornwall, UK

Ruth Davies Bristol, UK

Kenneth Capron, Maine, USA

Vesta Brownbill, Leicestershire, UK

Caroline Benham, Northamptonshire, UK

Claudia Reyes LLOYD, Middx., UK

Heidi Deboer, La Vergne, TN, USA

Samantha Shanks, Bristol, UK

Marla Kurtz, Toronto, Canada

Irene Mackay, Falkirk, Scotland

*Linda Jones, Wales, UK

Ian Casely, Powys, Wales, UK

Janie C Keary,Powys, Wales UK

Lisa Shaylor, Coventry, UK

Lisa Doran, Devon,UK

*Carol Olsen, Warrington, UK

*Bakhus Saba, Ontario,Canada

*Sherry Heppner, MB, Canada

*Ian Hatton, Manchester, UK

Sonia Edwards, Middx. UK

Chris Harding, Daily Sparkle, Totnes, UK

*Linda Skipper, Devon, UK

Gillian Hesketh, Lancs. UK

Ann Napolitan, The Long & Winding Road NY USA

*Jackie Smith

Darla Burton, Iowa, USA

Suzanne Linskaill, Edinburgh Scotland

Lisa Williams, Wales, UK

Samira Farhat, Tunisia, Africa

Anis ben Salem, Tunisia, Africa

Layla Chargui, Tunisia, Africa

Anne Dickens. Tasmania, Aus

*Kate Lewis, Chepstow, UK

*Gina Edwards, Conwy(Via Chris), Wales, UK

Julia Eagle, Cheshire, UK

John Westwood, Abergele, Wales, UK

Sebastien Fages, France Head of Ops,

*Sarah Jewel (Rowe), Cornwall, UK

Jan Inman, Essex, UK

Nicola Halewood Peers, Denbigh, UK

Tanya & Roger Pell, Forgetmenot Berks. UK

Michael Durose, Promem,Cornwall, UK

Kath Toms, Ivybridge, Devon, UK

Rhian Kiki Garvican, Nottingham UK

Caroline Dearson, Essex, UK

Noeline Jones, Australia

Rita Anand, Dementia Angels.org

Anna Tatton,

Shirley McGee, VA, USA

Teresa Noakes, Notts. UK

Maggie Fletcher, Staffs, UK

Karen Wheating, Dorchester, UK

Amanda Patrick, Wakefield, UK

*Verena Edgeworth, Bristol, UK

Jackie Roy, Daventry, UK

Julie Reddican, Abergele, UK (Olinda)

Gail Sonnesso,

Alex Morgan, Plymouth, Devon.UK

*Andrew Hughes, Olinda, Wales, UK

Jody Merenick, Wisconsin, USA

Theresa Manzardo, Seattle/Springfield Missouri USA

Christine Logan, W. Midlands, UK

Mary Anson, Crossroads Care, Cornwall, UK

Peter A Leussink, Austria

Larissa Dunnett, Upper Hutt, NZ

Heather Pearson, Southampton, UK

Gina Edwards, Conwy, Wales, UK

Jennie Morrison-Cowan, Sussex, UK

Sandra Hastings, Silverline, Newcastle upon Tyne UK

Linda Webb, Walton-on-Thames, UK

Patricia Eyre, Somerset, UK

*Christine Clifford, London, UK

Veronica Male, (Billingham) Northampton, UK

Paul Hamer, Devon, UK

Diane Carbo, NJ; USA.

*Ian Thomas

Emy Almeida

*Shannon Garner

Susan Kiser Scarff, Arizona, USA

Simone Bryan, Wrexham, UK

Tracy Pichardo, Barnstaple, UK

Kathleen Roberts, Wrexham, UK

Somaya, Egypt.

Cllr Lindsay Ward, Devon, UK .

Andy Powell, Bideford, Devon, UK

Julie Jones, Arizona, USA

Julie (Garner) Jones, Lytham St Annes, Lancs UK

Claire Paterson, Pencuik, Scotland

Lynda Henderson, NSW Australia

Angie Collinson and Steve, W Yorkshire, UK

Sylwia Rauch, Poland

Clarke Pollard, Naples, Fl. USA

Annette Brandstaetter, Solihull, UK

Jane Granger, Kent, UK

Renea Phenix, Florida, USA

Judith Chester, Guildford, UK

Ken Wong, Ontario, Canada

Jacklyn Pollock, Edinburgh, UK

Julie Sian Davies, Wrexham, UK

Peta Cunningham, Reading, UK

Steffi Frieser, Germany

Stefanie Lemmen, Nordrhein-Westfalen, Germany

Shannon O'Halloran, Hull, UK

Christine Phillips, Hartlepool, UK

Judy Alloway, Kingston, Devon

Rena McDaniel, USA

Helen Skuse, Torquay, Devon,UK

Margaret Field, Cheshire, UK

Angel Fedeline-Windsor, Dorset, UK

Michelle Willock-Watts, Devon, UK

Chloe Myers, Devon, UK

Caroline Grogan, Queensland, Aus

Maxine Bailey, Doncaster, UK

Victoria Lyons, London, UK

Julie Hayden, Berkshire, UK

Michelle Greenwood, Lancashire, UK

Anita Curley, Wales, UK

Stephen Corcoran, Liskeard, Cornwall. UK

Emily Skeffington, N Wales

*Sophia Colkin, Devon, UK

Helen Doel, Wiltshire, UK
Sue Moon, Wiltshire, UK

Linda Houston, Wiltshire, UK

Rosey Sanders, Cornwall, UK

Dawn Hargreaves, Bolton, UK

Debbie McEvoy-McBrias, Knowsley, UK

Gemma Woodworth, N. Wales, UK

Sallie Rutledge, Devon, UK

Lisa Evans, Tameside, UK

Deborah Moffat, Queensland, Australia

Martina Dennison, Eire.

Michelle Philips, Southend on Sea, UK

Stephanie Janka, Torbay Care Trust, UK

Caroline Starkings, Torbay Care Trust, UK

Ruth Ferguson, California, USA

Roger P. Byrom, Braunton, Devon, UK

Lyn Cheetham, Oxford, UK

Jean Shiner, Birmingham, UK (and Sue)

Karen Butler, Essex, UK

Truthful L Kindness, Mendocino,California, USA

Jeff Wicks, Cinnamon Care,Sri Lanka HofOps

Satoshi Ide, Japan.

Takayuki Maeda

Myrna Norman, Vancouver, Canada.

Joanne Mountjoy-Dixon, Thetford, UK

Jonathan Cohen, London, UK

Heather Gately, Dublin, Eire HeadofOps,

Hendi Lingiah, France

Jane Woodjetts, Seveoaks, Kent

Debbie Bode, Thetford, UK

Miranda Skinner, Michigan, USA

Bob Warnes, Norfolk, UK

Ian Lucas, N. Wales, UK

Sheena McBain, Norfolk, UK

Angela Downing, Cornwall, UK

Tracy Long, Coventry, UK

Roy Farthing, Norfolk, UK

Robert Bowles, Thomaston, GA USA

Foluso Oyegbesan, Kent, UK (emails only)

Joanne Newport-Rand, Florida, USA

Penny Dale, Dorset, UK

Brian and Leonore Norris, Cornwall, UK

Anita Bull, Lincolnshire, UK

Amber Sprague, Mn, USA

Joyce Toone, Lancashire, UK

Sabrina and James Thayer, USA

Gayle Everest, Gibralta. Head of Ops

Dave Prescott, Liverpool, UK

Liz Hartshorne, Yorkshire, UK

Ann Marie Lovejoy, W. Sussex, UK

Vicky Bannister, Wigan, UK

Kay Hudson, Milton Keynes, UK

Georgie Parfitt, Devon, UK

Paula Gratton, Surrey, UK

Alexandra Johnson, California, USA

Marie Flannery, Queensland, Aus.

Patty Swanger, PA; USA

Tracy Hubbard, Staffs, UK

Linda Cameron Deafenbaugh, PA; USA

Susan A Kimball, PA; USA

Bruce Barnet, New York, USA

Sharon DeBoever, Virginia, USA

Elizabeth E Royce, Florida,USA

Trevor David Wigley, USA

Cynthia S Bell, N Carolina, USA

Wayne Mesker, Ohio, USA

Debby Campbell Cloyd, Arizona, USA

Laura Brandstaetter, Solihull, UK

Nikki Trueman, (Moss)Derbyshire UK

Kate Thurtell, Devon, UK (300)

Graham Walker, Devon, UK

Sarah Rich, Devon, UK

Will Johns, Brighton. UK

Doug Seubert, Wisconsin, USA

Bill Prescottt, Bristol, UK

Heather Saunders, N.Hants, UK

Karina Visha, Derby, UK

Fran Watson, Derby, UK

Kim Barstow, Middlesborough, UK

Malcolm Bruce,

Ruth Doyle-Oasgood, Somerset, UK

The Bex Marshall, London, UK

Bexi Owen, Liverpool UK

Carolyn Shaw, Isle of Man

Dianne Wood, Flintshire, UK

Andy Barrett, London, UK

Kathy Woolfall, Connecticut, USA

Angie Woolfall, Cambs,UK

Edwina Hoyle, S Carolina, USA

Tom Bohlke, N Ayrshire, Scotland.

Danielle Stott, Manchester, UK

Phillip Hutchings, Devon UK

Lorraine Roberts, Devon, UK

Sara Rich, Devon, UK

Samin Chhetri, Nepal

Carolyn Shaw, Isle of Man.

Ceri Dyson, Devon, UK

Debbie Hammond, Staffs, UK

Sian Roberts, Wales, UK

Rhian Mai George, Wales, UK

Tracy Godden, Essex, UK

Amanda Martin, Devon, UK

Julie Reshad, Devon, UK

Dona Gondwe, Middx, UK

Jill Halstead, Norway

Nermine Habib, Egypt

Monika Liborio-Walker, Brazil

Brendah Chongo Chyapewa, Zambia, Africa

Pam Brunell, NC. USA

Regina Breen, Co Tyrone, Ireland

Marion Smyth, Lisburn, N Ireland

Hilde Seal, BC Canada

Cathie Borrie, Vancouver, Canada

Penny Bingham, Victoria, Australia

Jacqueline Crowther, Cheshire, UK

Manda Haworth, Powys, Wales

John Ormento, Massachusettes, USA

Barbara Leipow, NJ & Georgia, USA

Carol Smith, Wales, UK

Susan Rogers.Florida, USA

Reeta Ram, Watford, UK

Kayleigh Wood, Somerset, UK

Amanda Brookes, Wilts, UK

Alysia Adcock, Derbyshire, UK

Richard Hammond, Reading, UK

Kikelomo Laniyonu Edwards, Nigeria HofOps

Bola Agbaje, Oyo State, Nigeria.

Timothy Adegunle Seye, Ogun State, Nigeria

Damilola Omololu, Lagos State, Nigeria

Professor Aduke Adebayo, Osun State, Nigeria

Badaki Oluwatosin Felix, Ondo State, Nigeria

Seiya Van Someren Okieghazi, Bayelsa State, Nigeria

Tosin Olawuyi, Oyo State, Nigeria

Ayomide Olumide, Ekiti State, Nigeria

Isla Wilson, Hants. UK

Paul L Jansen, The Netherlands

Marie & Michael Langely, Victoria, BC,Canada

Kerry Fearnley, Torpoint, Cornwall

Dr Clive Acraman, Cornwall, UK

Simone Willig, Germany

Jasmina Lambergar, Slovenia HofOps

Gemma McDonald, Blairgowrie Scotland, UK

Linda Pine, Manchester, UK

Adam Woods, Merseyside, UK

Ruth Coward, Leicestershire, UK

Derek Fisher, London, UK

Nik Burgess, Cornwall, UK

Cym Downing, Launceston, Cornwall, UK

Janet Ashenden, S. Derbyshire, UK

Leonie Ashenden, S. Derbyshire, UK

Amanda Davidge, Cornwall, UK

Aarati Poudel, Nepal

Kathi Check-Maher, NJ. USA

Shirley Bannister Bolton, UK

Millie Rowland, USA

Ceri James, Devon, UK

Samantha Hatton, Hertfordshire, UK

Charles J Jaggers, South Wales, UK

Dr Adesola Odofin, Nigeria

Professor J A Ogunsheye, Nigeria

Professor Olusegun Baiyewu, Nigeria

Chief Mrs Leticia Laniyonu, Nigeria

Teslim Gafari, Nigeria

Professor Bolanle Awe, Nigeria

Susan Onuoha, Nigeria

Dr Charles Afolabi, Nigeria

Yolanda Ugochukwu, Nigeria

Katie Bowden, Birmingham, UK

Mary Ann Drummond, NC. USA

Leslie Simon, PA, USA

Myra Azzopardi, H of Ops Malta.

Iriri-Ishola Anthonia, Delta State, Nigeria

Hailey Richman, New York, USA YA

Jacqueline Daly, Leeds, UK (Ireland)

Michael Hrywniak, London, UK

Michelle A Hill, Wisconsin, USA

Robin Holmes, North Carolina, USA

Subha Ray, New Zealand

Lisa Rodriguez, Florida, USA

Connie Norby, Wisconsin, USA

Lynda Tickell, Cambs. UK

Allison Bourke, Beijing, China

Penny Madge, Torpoint, Cornwall

Carrie Peterson, Copenhagen, Denmark

Sam Cross, Plymouth, UK

Elizabeth Dunbar, Vancouver, Canada

Katie Bowden, Birmingham, UK

Jane Scott, Victoria, Australia

Narelle Dogan, Melbourne, Australia

Jan Zimmerman, Watertown, WI., USA

Natalie Dobson, Cumbria, UK

Sherry Berger, Arkansas, USA

Anna Platt, London, UK

Sheila Diete-Spiff, London, UK

Jan E Elias, Wisconsin, USA

Christopher James Hoult, Caernarfon, Wales

Robert Arsenault, Beijing

Karen Owen, N. Wales

Renee Smith, Sydney, Australia

Catrin Hughes, N. Wales

Ceri Whitten, N. Wales

Kirsty Hodkin, N. Wales

Joanne Hosking, Cornwall

Martha and Anna Hosking, Cornwall, UK ya.

Jane Sleeman, Cornwall, UK

Emma Jane Hardy, Devon, UK

Heather Bolderston, N. Wales

Tracey Owen, N. Wales

Ashling Newman, Galway, Ireland

Beth Covault, MI, USA

Bryan Cramer MI, USA

Brenda Reece, N. Carolina, USA

Janet McLean, BC, Canada

Christine Haworth, W. Midlands, UK

Sam Major, Bideford, Devon, UK

Lea Mason, Oxfordshire, UK

Marion James, TX , USA

Paula Stout, Manchester, UK

Susan Walker, Devon, UK

Ruth Ablett, Devon, UK

Neil Craig, GWR

Fiona Ambler, Berks, UK.GWR

Raymond Wilcox, Shropshire, UK

Kay Pahil, Birmingham, UK

Melissa Chan, Singapore

Alison Browning,

Tristan Holtger, WI, USA

Nicole Seberger, Iowa, USA

Vicky Beard, Illinois, USA

Vicky Zhang. China

Patrick Leese, Denmark.

Maria Fernanda Mandujano, Mexico

Debbie Lamberson Eastin, Oklahoma, USA

Kate Knapp, MN.USA

Deanna Breuker, BC., Canada

Kathryne Fassbender, WI., USA

Julie Anne Halliwell, Cyprus, UK H of Ops

Gabriela Matic, Glasgow, Scotland

Susanne Mitschke, Glasgow, Scotland

Patrick Renner, Glasgow, Scotland

Rogelio Arellano, Glasgow, Scotland

Debbie Lesperance, KS, USA

Jamie Theobald, Devon, UK

Tina Urquhart, Polyphant,Cornwall

Tony Stowell, London

Samantha Banks, Cornwall

Julie A Fleming, GA; USA

Gill Phillips, Devon, UK

Sarah Leadbetter, W. Sussex. UK

Ashma Devkota, Nepal

Lynda Cherry, UK

Milena Acraman, Cornwall, UK ya

Megan Payne, Cornwall. UK ya

Leah Hancock, Cornwall, UK ya

Maxim Hamley, Cornwall, UK ya

Helyn Glover, Sunderland, UK

Fiona Cameron, N Scotland, UK

Princess Khadijah Fedeline Windsor, BA Hons. Brighton, UK

Anil Pokharel, Lithuania.

Karin Heunes, Sth Africa

Jane D Ogilvie, Florida, USA

Sean Quinshuang, China

Carole Tribue, Spain

Hannelet Cloete, George, Republic of Sth Africa

Jo Dell, New Zealand

Sam Robinson, Lancashire, UK

Suzanne Bela, USA

Steven Singleton, California, USA

Daniela Manutius Forster, Hants, UK

Kathy Richardson, Bolton, UK

Eleni Andreou, Athens, Greece

Zach Gordon, Michigan, USA

Alison Hernandez, Devon, UK

Lisa Jane Masurier, Queensland, Australia

Ronald Fergy, Brent, London

Katie Corrick, Devon, UK ya

Enid Di Palmer, Riviera Afm. Devon, UK

Rachel Richards, N. Wales, UK

Lyn Stephens, Dorset, UK

Anne Dinnelly, Belfast, N.Ireland

Jon Webb, Westward Ho, N.Devon, UK

Jules Laverack, Northam, N.Devon, UK

Alison Henderson, Bolton, UK

Ayse Kucukkoylu, W. Yorks, UK

Paula Dunn, Bideford, Devon, UK

Kate Lewis, Chepstow, UK

Eileen & Neville Jackson, Queensland, Australia

Jenni Boydell Munster-Richard, Bolton, UK

Dr Krishna Prasad Pathak, Kathmandu, Nepal.

Shannon Lutmer. Texas, USA

Jacqui Eaton, Devon, UK

Stephen Lock, Devon, UK

Sandra Kelly, Keighley, Yorks. UK

Heidi Lund, Ringwood, Hants, UK

Amanya Luke Ronald, Jinja, Uganda.

Rosemary Hallett, N.Devon, UK

Alison Henderson, Bolton, UK

Nancy Lane, Sutton, MA. USA

Christine Collis, Letchworth, UK

Helen O'Leary, Australia

Jeanette Palmer, Illinois, USA

Tracie Sanders, London, UK

Rich Gardener, California, USA

Megan Randell, Surrey, UK

Lisa Battershill, Devon, UK

Regina Posvar, St. Lucia

Marlene Beards Wildman, W. Midlands, UK

Debbie Carder, N Devon, UK

Lorna Coulson, Devon, UK

Ramaa Subramaniam, India

Lyn Winter, N. Devon, UK

Matt Ray, N. Devon, UK

Countries around the world we are established in

46 COUNTRIES

AFRICA

AUSTRALIA

AUSTRIA

BANGLADESH

BRAZIL

CANADA

CHINA

CYPRUS

DENMARK

EGYPT

FRANCE

GERMANY

GIBRALTAR

GREECE

HUNGARY

INDIA

IRELAND (EIRE)

JAPAN

LITHUANIA

MALTA

MEXICO

MOROCCO

NEPAL

NETHERLANDS

NEW ZEALAND

NIGERIA

NORWAY

POLAND

ROMANIA

SINGAPORE

SLOVENIA

SOUTH AFRICA

SOUTHERN IRELAND

SPAIN

SRI LANKA

ST LUCIA

SWEDEN

TASMANIA

THAILAND

TRINIDAD & TOBAGO

TUNISIA

UK   (INC. WALES, SCOTLAND, ISLE OF MAN AND N. IRELAND)

UKRAINE

UNITED ARAB EMIRATES

USA

ZIMBABWE

THE END

OR IS IT ????????????????????

The Mountain They Call DEMENTIA ………………….

One day, one day soon, we will all look around and find ourselves finally on top of the mountain they call dementia. As we take in the view from the top we will notice others, many others, stood by us, side by side, looking at the same view, breathing the same clear air and feeling the weight of what seem like a lifetime lifted from our shoulders.

We will start to move closer to each other as we realise that we have all been in this together, then it begins, the first hug, then the second, the third until we are all hugging with relief, knowing at last a cure has been found and dementia banished forever. Smiles begin to erupt as wide as any ocean on earth just before the first teardrop falls, a teardrop of pure happiness and jubilation that begins a river, a sea , a tsunami of billions of tears wept by everybody. Tears of complete happiness and joy but also tears of relief.

Soon these tears of joy turn to tears of sorrow for all we have lost to this awful disease, for all they went through, their pain, their frustration and their anger at knowing that all they ever knew and worked for was being eaten away by this invisible devil. Suddenly, all will begin to realise how much of their own lives they have given, their time, their effort, their unrelenting patience and unconditional love, given without a thought and in a heartbeat.

Then, relief begins to wash over all as they now realise, all that anger, all that pain and all that frustration has been eradicated by the cure, and the walk to the top of the mountain the call dementia was all the time and love that they put in. As they stand and look around them, holding hands, together as one family, they know a new dawn has broken and life will never be the same again, but much better for all.

Printed in Great Britain
by Amazon

23439370R00126